BEYOND OBEDIENCE

Guidance and wisdom for all who are called to Mastery,
Ownership,
surrender, slavery, and service.

SlaveMaster & slave 7

Summer Sterling, Ed.

Table of Contents

INTRODUCTION

About Summer Sterling

My growing interest in Buddhism taught me without a doubt that ego is often my worst enemy. I often ran the dynamics of my surrender to my husband off the rails, "knowing" my way was the best way, and frequently required his needs to wait for a break in my schedule; after all, I had a lot on my plate, I reasoned. I was inconsistent, and constantly frustrated by what I saw as failure, or at the very least, something somehow lacking in myself. I knew what I wanted, but I continued to fail at maintaining it. I was happiest when in 24/7 surrender to my husband, so why did I keep fighting it? I *wanted* it. Yet, my damned ego kept rearing its pointy little head at the most inopportune times, telling me it might not be such a good idea, and to keep my obedience options open.

And so I found myself on the internet, poring through site after site to learn more about what I must be doing wrong, and searching for some solid answers on how this 24/7 lifestyle is successfully "done." But I knew I didn't need to read another blog post of the day-to-day mechanics of the M/s and D/s relationships out there. I don't care if I never read another post about removing stains from a Master's clothing or getting mold out of a Dom's shower grout. And you can bet I was sick to death of posts about the endless ease and beauty of submission. I wanted someone to step up to the plate and be honest about how challenging the lifestyle can be. Surely there were other slaves and subs out there who were frustrated, dog-tired, and as confused as I was about where they were going wrong. I wanted some solid answers. What I wanted most was some honesty.

The day I got into an argument with my husband about a decision of his that I hated, but a decision to which I submitted and still do, was the day I stumbled upon www.BornSlaves.com and numerous articles written by a man calling himself SlaveMaster. I could tell immediately that he had education, he had experience to back up what he believed in, and he demonstrated further credibility in the way he expressed himself. Let me tell you, this man can write. I checked out the BornSlaves blog, run by one of his slaves—slave 7— and was drawn to his wisdom and humility. I posed a few questions to him about my confusion and frustration. After receiving thoughtful replies, I read through countless articles and blog posts by SlaveMaster and slave 7, and I was hooked. I had "by accident" found people who called life exactly as they saw it, and were living accordingly.

I emailed slave 7 and said, "Reading what you write makes me feel as if I'm sitting by a quiet, peaceful stream. Have you and SlaveMaster ever considered writing a book?"

And here we are.

I know for a fact that I would make a terrible slave, and I can state with the utmost certainty that SlaveMaster would tell me it is because I was not born to be one. And this is one of the subjects you will read about in "Beyond Obedience" — the requirement of being *born* to such a life. Most important, you will read of his conviction that not only are slaves to live in absolute obedience, but Masters and Owners must also. Mastery and Ownership are not simply about issuing orders or having needs met. These individuals must respond to a call from the Universe or Spirit or The Great IT — whatever name you wish to attach — to live a life in obedience to ITs instructions and messages. And through obedience to the Master or Owner, the slave and those in surrender to others in turn obey the spirit. And so we come to learn that the lifestyle many are called to is not in and of itself about giving orders and hearing "yes sir," or, conversely, serving dinner, doing laundry and performing errands, but about a much higher calling, a calling from the Divine — a call that requires obedience from ALL who choose to listen to what the universe is requesting at any given time.

You will find the wisdom and guidance from SlaveMaster and slave 7 to be applicable to many walks of life. Whether you're a Master/Owner, a submissive/slave, or someone committed to a life of service or surrender, you'll be able to see yourself in the writing. For the sake of simplicity, however, the entities in "Beyond Obedience" are primarily referred to as Masters, Owners and slaves, and are most often referred to as male. It is tedious, to say the least, to try to list all possible combinations, and attempts to be all-inclusive at every mention can make for a rather plodding read.

Articles written by SlaveMaster are interspersed throughout and are in bold print. Comments by slave 7 are noted as such. I know you will find 7's writing to be especially thought-provoking and worthy of contemplation. For some, there may be confusion at first in his use of it, this slave, and the uncapitalized "i" when referring to himself. It is his and SlaveMaster's belief that this is appropriate for a slave. You will find a more lengthy explanation within the pages of this book.

I have never met SlaveMaster or slave 7 (although I hope to have the honor someday soon), yet I am emboldened not only by their connection, but also by their wisdom and instruction, which they share willingly and without charge to anyone seeking their guidance. I know I can speak for them when I invite you to join all of us who are sharing our experience while on a rare, alternative path. Please visit www.BornSlaves.com , and their new FetLife group at: https://fetlife.com/groups/111118.

About SlaveMaster
In His Own Words

In the late 70s, I visited my first adult bookstore and discovered a leather magazine filled with men riding motorcycles; wearing leather, and interacting with leather sex toys and restraints. I held that magazine up and, to my surprise and the surprise of everyone in the bookstore, yelled in shocked recognition, "Yes! Yes! I AM one!"

Until that day, I had been a dysfunctional heterosexual, but then, for the first time in my life, I knew who I was. And I faced a choice between being sexually functional, open and authentic with my new identity, or continuing my former "ideal" life with its considerable assets, enviable career and powerful political connections. I walked the street for hours with a heart frozen with fear. I decided to abandon the life I had so skillfully crafted, in exchange for a motorcycle to ride in cold, rainy weather, and a cheap studio in "that" part of town.

I found a family in a burgeoning leather community, and then immediately began to fear that I had become a dysfunctional homosexual. In the casual sexual atmosphere of the era, I discovered myself incapable of climax unless I felt both influence over and responsibility for my sexual partner. So, I desperately began perfecting the power dynamic demanded by my sadomasochistic sexuality. I initiated the clumsy process of learning how to find men who wanted to be tied up and whipped, by way of a dating ritual that included meeting at least once for a sober lunch or dinner to find out what my dates' interests really were. We openly discussed bondage and restraints, how often and how long they had worn a leather hood, and how often and with what results they had been bound, flogged or paddled. Even with all this preparation, I had experiences where men ran from the room as soon as I started to do something they had told me they loved.

With experience, I developed technical and psychological expertise. I could use hoods, blindfolds, floggers, tight restraints, ropes, tit and cock-and-ball torture devices, dildos and electrical stimulation devices, all without losing my partner's confidence or destroying their sexual excitement. I was consistently capable of facilitating entertaining, diverse and cathartic physical, emotional and even spiritual experiences. *I had figured out the magic combination to my sexuality.*

My sexual fetishes had seduced me into accepting a destiny of locating and empowering others to accept their destinies through a disciplined spiritual practice called "slavery," which employs the use of sadomasochistic devices. The myth of S/M is that the perfect pairing is a sadist— one who enjoys inflicting pain, and a masochist — one who enjoys pain. This is false. A true sadist only enjoys inflicting pain when there is no consent. Masochists are characterized by their need for control. Therefore, by their nature, sadists and masochists are mutually exclusive personalities.

The purpose of my practice is to produce spiritual evolution—permanent change, not simply an experience. Authentic spiritual growth never comes from experiences the ego can predict or control. So, to empower destiny, I create situations that go beyond the "safety" of S/M, and provide a powerful, efficient tool for focusing full attention on the present moment. When these devices are wielded with conscious spiritual intent and from a place of love, surrendering to their power simultaneously holds us in the present, fills us with love and teaches us how to embrace life on life's terms, without weakness.

Honesty is one of the results of this practice. When bound and restrained, the stimulation and power we feel finally free us to react in any way that is honest. When combined with the intention of love and power, that honesty can lead to levels of self-discovery that are unmatched by any other means.

My job is to give those who seek destiny the tools with which they can personally determine, assess, reject or accept as legitimate truth that which they learn. I don't dispense the truth.

Some prejudices can deny us the experiences that our soul requires to achieve integration. We forgo the life we have been created for because we fear what others might think. But our spirit doesn't care what anyone else thinks. It doesn't even care what we think, and it will never ask us what we want to do with our lives. It cares only about integrating every compartmentalized aspect of our lives into a unified, fully functional whole, capable of fulfilling our destinies.

It is our differences, if we honor them, which make each of us uniquely qualified to achieve our destinies. When we claim our normal gay life or normal lesbian life or normal heterosexual life, and then insist that we know what is true for us should also apply to everyone else, we are making the same mistake the religious right makes in demanding, "What's true for me is true for everyone." And if, in the resulting self-righteousness, we are avoiding a spiritual practice, we are cheating ourselves of the only life we can inherit: our own.

"Every comment I make comes from the perspective of My obedient position in life, which began with a defining moment in which I swore to never believe anything I wasn't willing to live by, and to live by everything I believe. When what I express has meaning to you, it is meant to have meaning. When it doesn't, then it's not yet meant to have meaning for you."

This book will only speak to whom it is supposed to.

Slave 7
In His Own Words

I grew up in suburban L.A., playing street hockey and body surfing with my two brothers and the neighborhood kids.

I grew up in poverty, with an alcoholic, drug-addicted, pothead father.

I grew up a child prostitute, so that my father could get the drugs he needed.

I grew up without church and religion, but with cult ritual abuse.

I started learning to play guitar at age 16 and started writing songs.

My 20s were a period of distancing myself from involvement in the past, of growing beyond it. Rock and roll was my vice, without the drugs and with only a little of the sex.

I had powerful desires to be slave.

My 30s were a period of facing the past and myself. I saw a psychotherapist for many years and was a member of a long-lasting men's recovery group for sexual abuse survivors. I came to even more deeply understand humans and humanity through a psychological lens, and saw all things spiritual and religious as being a kind of weakness, a lack of ability to see the hard truth, a denial mechanism.

My need to be slave did not dissipate. Still, I saw that need as something borne out of my childhood, that it was the result of nurture, not nature.

I had three significant partners over two decades, but never a Master of any kind. I never met one that seemed qualified to handle what I felt inside. I encountered writings online that made my cock hard and my heart pound and gave me my first encounter with Masters who were truly different from the gay leather crowd, one of which was SlaveMaster.

I came back to the writings of SlaveMaster repeatedly through the years and read somewhere in these writings that SlaveMaster believes a slave never has to do anything to find its Owner, that the Universe will just create the meeting when the time is right. That is when I knew He was crazy.

I gave up on ever finding a Master, and actually lost the desire to be slave at all. The desire seemed to vanish. I just stopped caring, and stopped wanting.

I read somewhere online that SlaveMaster had moved to Nevada, but I never lifted a finger to find him. Why should I? I knew he was crazy, even though I found him compelling.

Months later, I went to dine with a friend of mine, and one of his friends joined us. My friend said, "He's a slave." I said, "I know. I see that collar around his neck." My friend then said, "His Master is well known. Have you ever heard of a guy by the name of SlaveMaster? That's his Master."

My heart stopped. My breathing stopped. I had been brought into contact with SlaveMaster without any effort to do so. But I dismissed the idea of meeting SlaveMaster as I still believed He must be some kind of a nut. A few months later, however, I was invited to eat dinner with SlaveMaster and His slave. My first impression of SlaveMaster was of a man full of life and the love of life, and with lots of that love to share. This first impression was not wrong. SlaveMaster's first impression of me was that I was slave, but not ready to start slave development.

It took me a couple months to come to grips with the rebirth of the need to be slave that I was feeling inside, but I finally emailed SlaveMaster to schedule a talk about it. We talked for an hour about slavery in His hot tub while His mother sat in the living room waiting for us. (Yes, His mother knows all about her son and lovingly accepts Him for who He is.) A week later we had our first session, and it almost immediately felt clear that i belonged. Our second session was one month later, and it was then when i knew the slavery i had yearned for throughout adulthood was true and good and would become reality.

That weekend, i met my "self." The words coming out of His mouth were expressing points of view on goodness and the concerns of life that i had only ever heard myself say, at least in that manner. i was so stunned i wanted to pray. i was still an agnostic, bordering on atheist, but amazing things happened during subsequent sessions with SlaveMaster. i was sensing the Divine, but not from SlaveMaster, nor from His voice, for He was silent.

The Divine was coming directly to me. i was awakening. i was self-actualizing. i was what i always dreamed i was: not a fully independent human being, but one connected to another. And for me, that other is SlaveMaster.

All SlaveMaster ever does is give of Himself so that slaves may live the life they crave and need. He is love and stability on two feet, a rock for slaves to stand on — a giver, not a taker, and a Man who serves.

And this is joy and love, because this is who i am designed to be.

A Note to the Reader from SlaveMaster:

I have an academic background in science and am prepared to accept that one day all the "Rules of Life" can be explained through science. I don't think that day has come, and communication that puts everything into a complete perspective that doesn't use common words and accepted meanings would be incomprehensibly confusing. In the past, daytime was explained as being chariot races of the gods that begin each morning and end each evening. Now we theorize that it is a hydrogen fire instead.

My life wouldn't be one bit different if that chariot race was still the accepted explanation. Knowing the absolute, scientific, final truth about how things work isn't important. What is important to me is having a set of beliefs that is functional and efficient. They don't need to be ultimate truths, but they do need to be consistent and complete.

I have, therefore, selected modern beliefs and definitions to describe my "Mythology." It is a set of personal principles that forms a complete functional whole. I don't defend their final accuracy. No philosophy, spirituality or religion can be defended empirically. I do defend the functionality that allows operating from a sense of directed moral certainty. That's all I need.

I have found it important to accept that which applies now, and to allow my beliefs to change as I change, grow and mature. Defending what no longer works is a futile pursuit. I invite the reader to accept what works, reject what doesn't, and hold the possibility that at the right time in our lives each belief will serve a purpose.

WHO IS A BORN SLAVE?

The word "slave" has been used historically in a wide variety of contexts. It has been used to describe non-consensual, forced slavery, politically imposed slavery, a form of role play, a relationship usually with a "Master," as a practice, generally in conversation to imply something that is a drudge, and even to equipment which is triggered or controlled by other equipment, as in computer drives.

In the context of this book, "slave" and "Born slave" are used interchangeably to describe an internal, created characteristic that is present before genetic birth, and which is explored and discovered through life, then fully implemented in a moment which significantly marks who someone is authentically. That moment I call "Birth," because it is a change in the way the world and the "self" are viewed, and is also similarly associated with the drama of a genetic Birth.

The word "obedience" is referred to in this book in a very specific way, and is the same as "an alignment of the will." Obedience is not compliance which measures whether or not a task is completed. Obedience is not agreement in which an order is considered, reviewed, compared or assessed prior to accepting an order. Obedience begins when the response to any and every order is "Sir, Yes Sir" BEFORE the command is issued.

This rigorous understanding of obedience is necessary because compliance and agreement don't yield the same benefits or results. Any thought about how an order feels, whether or not it makes sense, sounds like a previous order, or any other comparison or assessment, is acceptable in compliance and agreement. Completion of an order is NOT done out of obedience, however, when any of that is present or has occurred. The task is accomplished, but the significant personal benefits that can produce Born slavery are denied.

A Born slave is a creature whose purpose is to be something more than human. Without personal experience, I suspect that what is true for men is also true for women.

Slaves are special creatures who:

Are capable of spending the rest of their lives without ever again performing an immoral act.

Are capable of unblemished honesty and integrity.

Have the courage and conviction to explore, discover, and, most important, live the truth, and nothing else.

Don't need excuses but, instead, do everything they should do, nothing more and nothing less.

Are capable of giving up the right to ever feel anger, to ever judge another, to ever disobey.

Are willing to live life instead of observe it.

Are willing to be the observed instead of the observers, to be the criticized instead of the criticizers.

Are so powerful they cannot act out of weakness under any circumstance.

Can feel and express another's love without concern for the consequences.

Are so pure, so developed, and so directed that they can live freely by another man's will, and have, nor want, any other will.

Are willing to experience anything their Owner wants them to so they will know the truth instead of only having heard about it.

Are willing to get over themselves and recognize that life isn't about them, it is about what they can do for the world, and that nothing else matters.

Can stand being extraordinary in all things, who don't want to settle for anything, or be any less than they can be.

Are as pure and refined, as dedicated, respected and revered as the finest sword in the hand of the finest swordsman in existence.

Are without limit or limitation.

Are of impeccable and unquestionable character.

Are as comfortable cleaning a toilet as giving a keynote speech to the United Nations.

Find as their only pleasure and enjoyment their ability to obey.

Are willing to never take credit for anything they do for the rest of their life because they know they ARE their Owner, and it would be stealing to take the credit.

Can participate in and expect miracles to happen to accomplish the orders they are given.

See miracles as ordinary because miracles are so much a part of their life.

Cannot feel pathological fear, nor anger, nor resentment, nor revenge, nor hatred, nor spite, nor vindictiveness.

Have the courage to give up their easily dispensable egos for a real life.

Can easily see everyone else's faults and limitations, and still love and respect them anyway.

Are not bound by the past, and are unconcerned for the future because they have the courage to live honestly in the moment, always.

WHAT IS BORNSLAVERY?

Bornslavery is a spiritual evolutionary benchmark. Language doesn't contain words that accurately or consistently define anything in the spiritual realm. Communication depends on having the same word represent the same meaning to everyone involved in the communication. Without any words to begin with, finding common understanding isn't possible.

The Birth benchmark of slavery is between a slave and the "Universe." I am a witness to the event, but do not confer Bornslavery. Unlike receiving a graduation certificate which confirms the successful completion of a set curricula, the granting at the special moment of Birth comes directly from whatever the Creative Intelligence is, and is granted based on ITs own criteria.

My responsibility is to provide slave development that is directed by the same intelligence that grants Birth. Every use of a physical S/M device is intended to grow the slave toward and through the moment when the benchmark is achieved. Development session after development session is required to present a slave with everything it must encounter, and force a slave, with willing consent, through what it needs to go through. There is no control over what has to come up, what has to be challenged, or what has to be empowered.

The Birth event occurs at a specific moment in time. It isn't a gradual process that gives any clues about when it is imminent. There aren't any road signs along the way that give any clue about how far a slave has come, how far it still needs to go, or what divergent routes might have to be traveled to get to the destined moment. The Universal Connection can be achieved during any development session and at any time during a session.

The singular, most fatal barrier to Birth is the desire to achieve it. I don't speak of Birth very often, and I don't describe Birth as an objective. Any conscious expectation or desire to achieve Birth absolutely prevents it from ever happening. In each of the more than half-dozen Births I have witnessed, in every case, the desire to achieve it was the final challenge to acquiring it. The slave had to convincingly conclude that it didn't care if it ever reached Birth before Birth was granted.

The consistency with which "desire" prevents achievement has confirmed a life lesson by which I feel obligated to live. Spiritualists have written that praying for specific things or results produces the greatest chance of never achieving what is prayed for. To ask for something confirms, over and over, that what we are requesting is absent from our lives. That thought of absence is the prayer that is being delivered. The alternative is to want only what is given, and to receive what is given as a gift, in gratitude. The slave protocol that requires a response of "SIR, YES SIR, THANK YOU, SIR!" as the response to any order, any discipline, or any question is the practice of this life lesson, and is crucial to Birth.

Birth occurs when we have accepted all of life's lessons as the Truth, and have become sworn to living by those lessons from recognition of how imperative it is to do so. The development of a Born slave has as its singular greatest priority providing an acceptance of the "Rules of Life" as they really are. I am never asked, nor do I ever expect to influence, what those rules are. My task is to provide the environment in which there is the opportunity and strength to experience them first-hand, in the presence of the mental tools needed to discern fact from fiction, interpretation, and wishful thinking, from objective reality. The stronger the tendency to create stories around everything that happens, or has happened in the past, the greater the challenge to move a slave to objective reasoning. Seeing everything as it IS, is a minimum requirement for qualifying for Birth. Refusal to accept things as they are is the underlying cause for rejecting Bornslavery.

I have observed Birth more than a half dozen times. I named the process "Birth" the first time I observed it because of the drama, trauma, emotion and dramatic change of paradigm that occurs during the process in a few short moments. So much happens so quickly that it is easy to see when Birth has occurred. There is no mistaking it for anything else. A few questions to the slave about what happened confirm what is observed.

I thought I knew all about Birth when I had witnessed it only once. With one example from which to draw my conclusions, it was easy to believe that any subsequent Births would be exactly the same. The second was very different from the first, and the third very different from the first two. Each Birth, in succession, was as different as the slave that experienced it. Now, with still less than a statistically valid number of observations, I can describe, at least, what was apparent and in common in each of the Births.

Adulthood is inherited. Emotionally, there is no formal Rite of Passage into adulthood in our culture. We begin our lives, and spend most of our lives thereafter, being told what is right and wrong, what we should be doing, and with whom we should be doing it. Our parents' influence is augmented by religious influence, modified by work influence, and strengthened by spousal influence. We walk through life being observers, watching for the reaction we get from what we do and say.

Adulthood is a feeling of an internal sense of wrong and right which allows an independence from what others think of what we are doing. We are free to become the observed instead of being the observers. We are free to do what our heart leads us to do, and to make a difference where our unique lives qualify us to make the most difference. Looking at the world through the eyes of a child becomes unnecessary and unproductive.

The spiritual world becomes real. It has been said that most of us reflect the belief that we are physical creatures having a spiritual experience during this life. Our words, our body language and our actions make what we feel transparent to an objective observer. Birth confirms an acceptance that we are spiritual beings merely having a physical experience on this earth. Viewing our behavior and purpose from this perspective changes our decisions, motivations and life connections. Nothing that happens is about us. Everything that happens has a meaning and a purpose, and often contains an opportunity and a lesson.

Dedication to obedience is confirmed. When we examine the lives of those we think have discovered their destinies, it is easy to see they have an internal obedience that supersedes any other influence in their lives. We all attempt to trick "fate" into believing we are obeying enough that we can get the benefits. We try to give to get, and hope we can get away with it, without having to "buy into" swearing our lives to obedience. Birth presents knowledge that obedience is our connection to the source of what we are to do with our lives. Don't obey, and the channel is closed. Obey, and for so long as we do, the channel that directs our decisions, our pursuits, our achievements, our relationships and our passions remains open and constant. Knowing replaces believing. Removing all doubt about the possibility of ever disobeying provides confidence and conviction.

There are other observations that were common among the Born: Laughter. Seeing how silly it was to struggle against accepting life's simple Truths. Sadness: From recognizing all the effort that now feels wasted, from struggling against the inevitable. Disappointment: Knowing, finally, that the uphill battle was to the top of a mountain that never existed, but which felt so important and real while being climbed. Joy: The relief that what felt like giving so much up was actually giving nothing up, and inheriting the purpose and meaning that had prevented enjoying life and had created the feeling that something was missing.

Birth is as unique as the slave that experiences it. Wanting Birth stops it from happening. Wanting to give Birth, instead of the environment in which it can occur, compromises the integrity needed to provide it. Birth is real. Birth is worth achieving. Stop demanding it, and, instead, accept your created purpose, and Birth becomes the natural result of being alive for those destined to be Born.

ACCEPTING WHO WE ARE

An Article by SlaveMaster

Two of the most overwhelming challenges all humans are faced with are identifying who we are, and then accepting who we are. Whether Owner, Master, slave or anyone else, the challenges are equally great. In this group [BornSlaves], we are relating only to those whose lives are defined by who they are, and the associated title they claim. An Owner always IS who someone is. There is no alternative. Masters and slaves might be equally born to BE either Master or slave. Or, Masters and slaves might be born to have their mastery or slavery as only one more thing that they do, just like being a carpenter or fireman. Either way, we either ARE our roles, or these roles are only what we do.

Owners, along with the Masters and slaves, potential Masters or slaves, or those who belong to this [BornSlaves] group, know somehow that these titles are more than a profession, hobby, or just another characteristic of who we are.

The first challenge of identifying who we are is easy for some, and extremely difficult for others. Everyone comes to the self-realization in their own unique way. Along the way, a lot of things seem true for a while, but through exploration and the experiences gained, we let go of those old beliefs and move on to new beliefs and new self-images. We all start with our egotistic self-image and the beliefs that allow our ego's control.

We also start out with average descriptions of who we are. From the moment we understand a language, we are taught what is expected of us. Those expectations are always within the very limited confines of acceptable human behavior. This is how we are controlled and socialized.

Here among the [Bornslaves] group, we are exploring becoming extraordinary. All of the arguments that apply to average human beings belong with discussions of average people. The movement to becoming spiritually mature involves relinquishing average human logic in deference to Divine logic.

We don't define life. We can only discover life. When we quit trying to become what we're not, often after exhaustion, we can accept who we are. That takes great courage and sometimes great pain. It is never without cost.

As average citizens, if we enter a burning building to retrieve a fire victim, we are considered heroes. Our egos love being heroes. That's what the ego strives for. If, however, we claim ourselves to be a fireman, from qualifying to do so, we no longer have the option to go past anyone in a burning building. We are then doing the minimum expected if we go to extraordinary means to retrieve someone from a fire. We are disciplined, if not fired, if we fail to do what would have been heroic for an average citizen, but what is only the fulfillment of minimum responsibility when titled "Fireman."

The courage to claim who we are is one of the greatest acts we will ever perform in our lifetime. We must overcome our natural cowardice when we claim the responsibility of who we are. We must permanently give up the opportunity to be considered heroic from the average egotistic perspective. We must give up being average and become unsung heroes. My grandmother used to say, "Anything we do that others know about, we shall never be credited with."

When we recognize we are meant to lead or direct others' lives, we are accepting a deep and moral responsibility. Every order we issue must carry with it moral responsibility for that order. A Master's ego would rather have His slave remain egotistically responsible, because then the Master doesn't need to be. It's cheap and easy to issue an order that we expect the receiver to remain responsible for accepting and obeying.

Courage is being qualified and willing to accept full responsibility for our orders. We are no more beneficial than a leather "Hints From Heloise" without the associated responsibility. All the platitudes about human dignity, intelligence and rights make great prose, but are nothing more than excuses to use and abuse, to the extent that another will accept our commands. Everything remains "their fault" because it was made clear they must think for themselves.

Issuing orders that are refutable is what every two-year-old does naturally. The child indiscriminately demands everything it wants and the parents' agreement with the orders is what protects the child from receiving more than it should have. The child takes no responsibility for anything demanded. The child doesn't need to, because the parents do.

Issuing irrefutable orders is what matters, what makes a difference, and what requires timbre, character, courage and strength. No child is capable of taking responsibility, so the parents must. Anyone who claims to command others, however, must take adult responsibility and not demand that the receiving slave carry the responsibility for acceptance. Making demands on another who must carry the responsibility for what is demanded is no different than the act of a demanding child.

The evolutionary purpose of every One who takes real responsibility, regardless of their title, is to find moral certainty. That means knowing for sure what to do. Until we have moral certainty, we are still conducting the demanding acts of a child. Moral certainty only comes from identifying, developing and maintaining a direct connection to the "Source" of all intelligence. The nature of that intelligence can be viewed differently by each, but acceptance and connection with IT is the critical essence of moral certainty.

Slaves are created without the capacity for moral certainty. Their connection is through us. If we don't have a morally certain connection, we can't give a slave theirs. We can't give what we don't already have. If a slave is capable of finding its own moral certainty, then it has no business pretending to be a slave. Slaves are not weak creatures who seek a co-dependent life to avoid developing their own morally certain connection. Slaves are potentially the strongest creatures of all of us.

It is in slaves' nature to only find the connection that allows moral certainty through their destined Owners. That's what draws them to us. If not for this reason, then we are only enabling some weakness or pathology that would be better cured through professional help.

Admittedly, moral certainty is an advanced human state. Most don't even hope to achieve the connection required in their lifetimes. The invitation to this group [BornSlaves] touches the part of you that knows there is something more, something beyond what humans can understand egotistically.

Our challenge here isn't to maintain our human egotistic identification and pride, not to discourage others from going beyond being average, but to surrender to our adulthood. Our task is to passionately proclaim our search for obedience, which, when found, defines all spiritual adulthood.

There are men and women in this [Bornslaves] group who have paid heavy prices to know who they are and to become who they are. We can learn from what they have gone through. We can save effort by knowing what they used to believe before they found and accepted the Truth. These people deserve and have my respect, none more than slaves, who also suffer societal denigration of their titles.

There is a law of life that we cannot give away what we don't have. Until we have self-respect, we can't give it to others. Whenever we find it difficult to give respect, we must examine the deficit of self-respect we find in our own lives. Naming as arrogant those who have the courage to claim their roles in life is such an average thing for the ego to do to justify not claiming one's own role in life. It is so much easier to maintain the chance to become heroic by claiming no title, thereby avoiding the responsibility that would come with such a claim.

Maslow told us that anything worth doing well is worth doing poorly until we learn how. None of us begins at "perfect." We all take small, stumbling steps while we learn to do what is extraordinary. We are measured in life by whether we encourage and facilitate those steps, or whether we mock and discourage them. That's what being either part of the problem or part of the solution is all about.

Another law of life is that we are either growing or dying. In each moment, we make decisions that determine which is happening. We have the collective potential here to become the most alive creatures on earth.

My thanks to all of you who are doing just that.

Additional Thoughts on Acceptance:

SlaveMaster:

All of us grow up with dreams of who we want to be. Some of those dreams are our own, and many are those given to us by our religions, our parents and our peers.

Most of our lives are spent in the pursuit of what is expected of us, and that we have accepted as being our own. To accept slavery is to give up all those personal dreams in exchange for the reality that obedience is all that a slave has a right to. That is a much harder reality to accept than that of being someone's victim.

I sense in many of us an embarrassment that we aren't at a "higher" level. That's like being embarrassed to not be in the sixth grade while still in the fourth. I once had a particular slave who when with Me could only talk about how much it wanted to be elsewhere in exotic places. When in those places, it always wrote back how much it wanted to be with Me. Never satisfied, always wanting to be where it wasn't.

Wherever we are is where we should be.

slave 7:

This slave accepted the following as a given in life: When one lives true, one will be satisfied. From a place of clear acceptance, jump into the river and let it take you.

The lesson for this slave was that life is not about doing. It is about accepting — accepting what life brings, accepting what one has within oneself, accepting lack of control, accepting that our thoughts are gifts and not our own creations, etc. The "doing" in life becomes the explicit acceptance and carrying out of orders.

Authenticity
(In the Extreme)

SlaveMaster:

Our drive to be happy is a search for being authentic, finding and being who we are created to be. Who we are will always be about what we can do for the world, and not what we can do for ourselves. The only reason to have any capacity is to influence the world according to the Universal plan.

slave 7:

It has been mentioned that living with SlaveMaster must be intense, but this morning 7 told SlaveMaster that 7's only thought is that perhaps 7 could be too intense a slave for SlaveMaster. SlaveMaster merely smiled and ordered that his slave "be all the slave that it is and that I need it to be," which was no surprise to 7. No slave can be "too slave" for SlaveMaster.

This slave believes that we live with models that work for us, that help us understand as best we can. Indeed, people often try to create the model, or reality, that they wish for themselves, or hold on to one given us during upbringing, but this doesn't work. Rather, we are pulled, or forced, by the reality within us toward whatever that reality is. Parents and social upbringing provide a model for us to live with, but often people need to break free from that model. Just being gay forces people to break free. Just wanting a life other than the one our parents want for us forces us to break free. Then, a new model is created or uncovered, only to be discarded or amended as the individual continues to grow emotionally, psychologically, spiritually.

Very few people, if any, would create a reality that made themselves slave. Rather, being slave makes us give up the models that society provides — and that we may want to live up to — in order to find one that matches what we know to be true and real within ourselves. People destined to be slave more often than not go to their slavery kicking and screaming, as you well know. Is the new model that matches our inner reality the real and true model of reality? It is for that individual at that time. Growth is allowing oneself to go from one model to the next, with new experiences, and new lessons learned. Somewhere along the line, or perhaps at many points along the line, one must take that leap of faith that the direction and the model are right, or at least the best one can do. Then, at a more ultimate point, one may be able to say what Joseph Campbell said: "I don't have to have faith. I have experience."

Follow what you know to be the truest within you, that which gives you joy or bliss, that which makes you feel centered and most real or authentic. Then, old modes of thinking will drop away and new ones will take their place. Take the leap and have the experience. The first response that comes to this slave is that only you can know what is the truest within you, only you can identify your bliss, and only you can know when you are centered, real, and authentically you. And only you can know when and how to take that leap of faith. The leap of faith itself is what lets you know you are moving in the right direction. Or, possibly, if you haven't taken a leap, then you are not moving. Taking a leap requires not knowing for sure in advance and giving up the sense of control you want to hold onto. Experience, internal movement, landing, confirming, and then moving on again.

And no doubt some are just pushed over the edge and forced to leap. In other words, just go for it. If you see the precipice and a possible landing, then take the chance and learn from the leap, wherever you may fall. You have the strength to pick yourself up, and many others will support you.

The strength comes from the feeling of truly being your authentic self and therefore "connected" to the heart and the Universe, of knowing that the motivations for any action are not based on concerns of the ego, that they come from some place beyond ego awareness such that you know you cannot take credit for them. Somehow, seeing/hearing/knowing the right thing to do just comes to you, as does strength due to confidence and moral certainty.

The truth is that when we do everything for the authentic self, we automatically do everything for others. When a slave totally honors its slave self and does everything for that slave self, it automatically does everything for its Owner. Thus, a selfish adherence to one's authentic self is at the same time the most giving a slave (or person) can be. And thus the freedom and lack of victimhood in slavery. Be totally who or what you are, and that is the best service you can be to anyone.

For those who have lived to know, accept and become who they really are, looking out at the world reveals billions of people who are extreme in their distance from their own authentic selves.

SlaveMaster does not allow loopholes and wiggle room away from what is real and true, and this makes many very nervous. What He does allow, or insist upon, is an avenue to your own heart, your true self, and your innate needs and desires. In this, He is extreme.

The goal in life is to grow to be ourselves (to be useful), not to remain or become what somebody else wants us to be (to be used).

BDSM

SlaveMaster:

Only those who are authentically Master/Owner or slave will ever find their evolution into the spiritual through BDSM. For those for whom it is not a created and authentic pursuit, BDSM will remain a part of their lives serving as entertainment, or more, that benefits their lives, but not the path of their life.

If you want to know how to "break" a slave, that's easy. Take anyone off the street, instruct that person to begin using S/M devices on the slave, and when the slave objects, keep right on going. It's that easy. Those qualified to develop others use the S/M device to transmit the Owner's Love and Power. No other intention or purpose can be allowed nor sought. Love and Power is the only environment that will grow a slave.

No one should ever pick up a device until that person knows what they want to accomplish. Breaking, hurting, power-exchanging, entertaining and humiliating are objectives, but have nothing to do with the best interest of the slave. These objectives have only to do with egotistic need of the physical S/M giver.

So, what do you want to accomplish? Every S/M session answers the question. Breaking, hurting, or humiliating doesn't accomplish anything. Go break a glass. Simply drop it on the floor. How is life any better now than it was before the glass was broken? Until we know what we want to accomplish, until accomplishing our objective is worthwhile, and until we are qualified to accomplish what is worthwhile, we are still exploring and developing. When your answer is "I want to empower My slave in the best interest of My slave," then use physical S/M to transmit your Love and Power. Nothing less and nothing more.

slave 7:

Every Owner/Master-slave situation is different. This slave has heard of Masters who use no S/M at all, and other Masters who use quite a lot. The real point is that the Owner or Master should know that each slave is different and then also know the right kind and amount of BDSM to use on each slave so that the slave gets exactly what it needs.

Also, it is indeed true that the more the slave's brain or ego is out of the way, the less "pain" it feels. As SlaveMaster has stated, when in a "pure slave state," a slave feels no pain.

Many abuse survivors who are also into BDSM come to believe that their BDSM needs (not necessarily slavery needs) come from their abusive pasts, and they learn to live with it, to love it, to see it as a part of themselves. In short, they just go with the cards they have been dealt, being better able to do so via the clear awareness and acceptance of their pasts. This slave came to believe, however, that it would have gotten into BDSM regardless of its abusive past, just because it is an explorer. But the whole question is moot, really, for there is no way to know. It is the age old nature vs. nurture question. This slave, via experiences it believes to be truly Spiritual, sees that its life has been managed by the Universe so that it is exactly what it is now.

This slave has never sought to be broken. Rather, it has always sought to be nourished and nurtured, to be connected to another so that it may live its life fully. For a slave such as 7, its Owner is its God, and Gods have the power to grow things. Mere men have the power to break.

BDSM activities can allow a slave to practice enduring and seeing things through to the end, which can then be transferred to real life out in the world. Routine paddling keeps the slave mindful that the butt is Master's butt and not its own, and Master can do what He wants with it. This slave feels it is good to look at the big picture. Paddling is only one part of its slavery, and slavery is not a thing that allows picking and choosing the parts you like.

BECOMING AN OWNER
An Article by SlaveMaster

The question is, why would you want to be an Owner?

The only reason that I have personally accepted being Owner is because I have no reasonable choice. It is my life and my destiny, and I wouldn't wish the job on my worst enemy. Nor would I wish on that enemy what it takes to gain the experience needed to provide slavery to someone. Until it is clear there can be no choice, I can't see why anyone would accept the assignment. It has no perceived personal benefits. It has to be only about serving the Universe. It allows for no time out and for no personal options. Once an Owner, that's who and what you are.

When you're a Master, you can have a slave who can provide service in any way that meets your needs. A Master "pays" for that service through His responsibility for His slave's life. As a Master, a man can exchange His responsibility for the benefits of having a slave unselfishly serve Him. There are no additional benefits that come from owning a slave. But, the added responsibility is without limits.

Being an Owner is without limitation, either in time, effort, or level of responsibility. When someone decides to be an Owner, He is committed for life to the best interests of the slave for the rest of His life. There is no identifiable reason for wanting to be an Owner, unless being an Owner is someone's destined purpose. The need to be Owner can come only from that deep, spiritual, immutable purpose. Any other motivation will quickly wilt with time.

Further, one outcome of becoming someone's Owner can be the need to assign the developed slave to someone else, geographically separated from you. When you are sworn to the best interests of a slave, then no selfish motivation can be exercised against the slave, including forcing it to live with you. Your investment, even if successful, is likely to walk out the door. The slave needs to fulfill its destiny; what else can it do? An Owner's destiny is to ensure that the slave's destiny is fulfilled. What else can He do?

Slave development is somewhere between difficult and impossible to accomplish when a slave is living with its Owner. The requirements for being slave are serious, often overwhelming. The need to examine some very difficult issues over and over dictates the slave have private time away from the Owner. An Owner cannot grant "time out" for a slave living in His presence, because that would pollute and destroy the Owner/slave protocol that is necessary for Birth. Once the chance of Birth has been removed, then there can be no potential for Ownership, and the whole process becomes moot. At that point the chance for the Owner's return on investment becomes zero.

A very good Master is one who loves, cares for, and feels a soul connection so great with His slave that He wants to give that slave its destiny of slavery. An Owner must create and maintain a life where emotionally and physically the slave's best interest outrank any personal or private selfish needs or motivation. There are human limits to investing everything in a single slave while generously making every decision to support what is best for the slave. There is a natural conflict between having all of a Master's personal needs and interests met by a single slave whose needs and interests must come before HIS own. If I have a need the slave isn't ready to provide, yet demand MY need be met anyway, the result could easily be a serious loss of trust, and retardation of the slave's development. An Owner cannot satisfy any personal need which isn't motivated by the slave's needs above all else.

What is an adequate motivation for being an Owner? The motivation must be that the Owner's purpose can only be satisfied with talents found in others. That purpose has to be achievable only when another performs the required actions on His behalf and for Him. The purpose must require that the action be performed where the Owner cannot be. That purpose must be the Owner's destiny. Any other motivation is insufficient. Being an Owner is a lifetime commitment, a commitment made to many, not just one slave. That is a lot of commitment to carry.

Another requirement is the number of slaves who must be developed as an Owner. Being an Owner is not a one-slave prospect, any more than building automobiles is a one-car project.

Providing a slave's destiny involves accepting the way life works. Statistically, that is impossible to determine from a single observation. There need to be many who are pursuing their slavery, many who have quit, many who have made it. The mix provides the experiences necessary to become informed and capable, to become qualified to be an Owner. And, being a destined slave isn't about having a monogamous relationship. A slave's special destiny has only to do with being available for the world, and to serve it. It isn't a private affair. It is a very public affair.

When someone attempts to become Owner to only one slave, then He is putting all His eggs in one basket. The Owner knows the slave must be free to leave at any time. The Owner has to be willing to invest all the unselfish effort, time and emotion required to supply unlimited direction, with unqualified dedication to empowering a slave's Birth, and life. How can an

Owner act only in the best interest of the slave when there is no one else to satisfy His needs?

When we know that we are placing all our bets on one person, we try to compromise, to make adjustments, to convince a slave to continue its slave development even when that isn't in its heart. We reduce the requirements and protocol required to allow for its slavery. The feeling of being left alone without the person in whom we have placed all our love, investment, and expectations prevents us from acting in the best interest of that slave. We are free to act in the best interest of another only when our own needs are not dependent exclusively upon that one other.

What is the advantage to being an Owner, when you could put your effort into, and find your rewards from, being a Master? The only answer must be that you are drawn to it, that you must be Owner to feel your satisfaction and happiness in life. Few ever ask about being an Owner. If, however, you do feel compelled to give your life to the life of slaves, there is a lot to consider.

Some humans are created with a singular soul, each with their own purpose. Those each independently find, pursue, and implement their individual destiny. Some are created as a set, to share the same soul. In that set are one Owner and the slaves who were created to share that singular soul. The Owner must see His slaves as a part of Himself, no more and no less than He is, because that's the truth. He is so much the same person as His slaves that He is morally responsible for everything they do, once they have accepted and achieved their obedience, their destiny, their Birth and their authentic life.

The Owner must have gone through His own discovery of destiny. He must have ended up in a position where He is permanently committed to being the Owner of the soul that is shared, and without any option to abandon it. Then, a permanent oath must be sworn to the Creator— the Source of life— that the Owner will act in the best interest of His slaves, without exception or limit, regardless of the effect on the Owner.

When your purpose, destiny and happiness are what you have prayed for, then you must be given experiences that are so traumatic that you would never consider abandoning your role. Any less, and the Universal Intelligence can't and won't trust you to do your job. Your obedience to the Ultimate Wisdom has to be more complete than that required of any slave. The Universe can't be tricked, so Birth will never be granted unless the Owner can be trusted by the Universe, and is therefore qualified to perform His destiny.

The Owner must develop all the techniques necessary to support the intention of giving the parts of His soul the experiences they need to accept not only the moment of Birth, but also their destiny. An Owner's destiny cannot be completed without fully developing the parts that belong to Him.

Developing others to their destiny introduces an Owner to being set up as the object of all the anger and disappointment and betrayal that a developing slave must experience to know for sure what its destiny is, and to accept that destiny. While you are developing a slave out of love and a completely unselfish motive, the developing slave will have to treat you like an enemy. An Owner is the worst enemy the ego will ever experience. The Owner must be the chronic, unrelenting enemy of the ego, or the ego will win and the soul will lose. No one has ever accepted his/her destiny while the ego is still important in his/her life.

When the Owner is the most loving and accepting, the prospective slave can be the most hateful, disrespectful, ungrateful, resentful, and combative. Every time the ego tries to entice you as Owner to anger, you most need to be ready to express unqualified love for the developing slave. If your image and position matter the least bit egotistically, you won't be there to provide the support the developing slave needs. Fail to be there, and you can never be an Owner.

The slave's ego will try to attack when you have the least time to deal with it, or when you are the most fatigued. The slave's ego becomes destructive and creative as the egotistic desperation grows. The more willing and open the Owner is about explaining all the things that a slave never needs to know about its slavery, the more vulnerable He becomes. Questions are asked just to find somewhere to attack. A slave doesn't need to know anything about anything except obedience to become slave. Everything else is unneeded and unnecessary. The only real value the information has is to the slave's ego that feels it must survive supreme and complete. The Owner only remains willing to answer to let His slaves know there is an answer and a reason for everything, which assures His continuing vulnerability.

As the superfluous ego's questions are answered, the slave's ego learns what the Owner's weak points are. The slave's ego uses the information it has acquired to become more divisive, and to implement its fits at the most effective time. And remember, there are several slaves with whom you are dealing at the same time, not just one.

If your time, effort or energy have to be under your control, you can never be Owner. Slave development doesn't occur at "convenient" times, it occurs when it isn't convenient at all.

No one can be turned down who honestly wants to develop its slavery. It would be playing God to decide who could have their destiny, or not. There can be no concern for age, looks, body type, or any other consideration other than the real potential that they might be your slave. Your personal reaction to a potential slave can have no bearing on whether or not you will willingly dedicate your life and love to each potential slave for the rest of your life. If personal independence matters to you, if you feel the need to decide who you like and who you love, being an Owner can't be your life.

As with any destiny, nothing you want matters. When we accept our destiny, we are accepting that we will ONLY do the Universe's work. We can't work both for the Universe and for ourselves. It has to be one or the other. Unless the Universe can trust that you will never again try to work for yourself, it won't allow you to become an Owner, and IT won't give the success of Birth, life and destiny to any slave. IT won't qualify you to be Owner.

For some, what might be the hardest of all is that slave development must be given without any expectation or intention to ever get anything out of the development process. The entire experience must be given as a pure gift. Over and over, and without limit, the gift must be given through the S/M and through love, and through spiritual direction until the slave is finally developed. Then, the Owner must take responsibility for the slave in every area in which it obeys, and moral responsibility for everything the slave does for the rest of its life, still given as a gift, without any recognizable benefit to Himself. Further, there can be no expectation nor limitation that the slave would need to live with nor serve its Owner directly, even after Birth. The mode must be unselfish, unselfish, and unselfish.

Some slaves who consciously achieve their slave destiny will be assigned to serve another as their

Master, and might not ever serve their Owner directly. After an Owner suffering all the effort and indignity, the slave could need to serve someone else, or serve somewhere else, walking out with all the resource you have invested. Furthermore, it is then also the Owner's responsibility to teach, advise, and direct the Master to whom the slave is assigned, or any others who come into the slave's destined life. Responsible Masters will also need the Owner's help to accept and execute the responsibilities the Master has for the slave who has been assigned to Him.

Just like a parent, an Owner is a spiritual parent, and remains responsible for all the direction needed through life. Where it lives, with whom, or what it is doing never relieves the need to make a slave's life complete, as a gift, without any expectation of personal benefit.

Still want to be an Owner?

The development process itself takes from months to years. The responsibility to the slaves' Masters, or any others of significance, never ends. The Born slaves need to be connected with from time to time to assure that their slavery continues to grow. Everything becomes more and more demanding, never less.

There is no divorce, and there is no way out. Once in, always in. The Universe can't be tricked, and IT can't be lulled into forgetting about us. We can't pretend to be permanently committed, then change our mind. IT has the resource to assure that everything continues as IT intends. When it wants a web page, that's what it gets. When it wants "Path of the Obedient Heart" retreats, workshops, presentations, seminars or personal one on one time, that's what IT gets, regardless of the effort, the exposure, the resource required; regardless of the inconvenience, regardless of the potential for criticism, regardless of its impact on any personal time, regardless of other commitments, and regardless of how you feel or what you would like to do.

If after knowing this you are still interested, then it is about getting spiritually clear yourself, and learning how to discover and enforce the Truth. An Owner must know that He has no black spot on His soul, because it will infect all of the soul, and the Universe won't allow that. IT controls the infection by refusing to grant Birth, by refusing destiny, and by denying the purpose of our efforts.

Birth, the conscious acknowledgement of destiny, is granted only by the Universe. There is no way to fudge or compromise the process. The Owner's obedience to the Universe, the spiritual world, and each order must be absolute. All egotistic motivation and intention has to be ignored, forever. Each potential and Born slave takes first priority in the Owner's life. Personal time is what is left over only after the primary responsibilities are taken care of.

There have to be several experiences, and even more failures, to learn what must be done as an Owner. When you have given your heart, and life commitment to potential slaves, they can still run out on you, usually for a lack of honesty or courage. Over and over they walk off with your heart, even when you know they are a part of you. Being emotionally thrown off the horse, you have to keep getting up again, and remain prepared to get right back on the emotional horse that just threw you off.

With all the gifts you give in love, time, attention, and expertise, they react in disrespect and anger at the One who wants to, and is the only one qualified to, give them their life, their destiny and their happiness. And it never ends. The Owner becomes the target for all their negative energy, and the Owner must invite it, because it is honest and necessary to their development.

Emotionally you are always exposed, and you have to learn to be more and more vulnerable. If you cut yourself off from any emotion, then you can't transfer your heart, your love, and your power to another part of your soul, and you can't give what is necessary to empower either their development or their destiny.

Being an Owner is a thankless job. The young and the pretty aren't interested in anything as serious as authentic slavery. You have to love everyone that comes into your life, and have no right not to give that love. The more you do, the more you have to do. Once you figure out how to do some aspect of the development process, the Universe raises the bar and forces you out of your comfort zone again, to learn something new, doing something even more uncomfortable. No matter how much you do, it is only the minimum required. There is no glory to bask in, and no one applauding any of the effort.

The most you can ever expect is an occasional kind word, and you can't be vulnerable to being flattered by it, because then you are vulnerable to being hurt when criticism is received, and, most important, will begin to compromise your integrity to attempt to gain the flattery once again.

There is no one in the world that you can talk to about what you are going through, so you are alone with your feelings. There is no one from whom you can get advice. There is no one who can be your close best friend. Most in the world can't even understand what you're doing after you have explained it to them, and few in the world are even interested in listening to the explanation.

Ultimately, our lives are about doing what we were Created to do. If you are an Owner, your connection to life, to love and to the world will come only from

qualifying for and living the destiny you have been assigned.

Nevertheless, there are those who are destined to be an Owner. If you are one of them and you want to be an Owner, let me know. I'll help you as I can, and I'll bless you every day for trying.

Additional Thoughts on Becoming an Owner:

SlaveMaster:

I see the role of a Master to be diametrically different from an Owner. I'm aware that most use Master and Owner interchangeably despite their dramatic differences.

What ultimately defines Born slavery can only occur when there are both a qualified and willing owner who will take full responsibility and a qualified and willing slave who will give full obedience. One (an Owner) finds obedience personally and individually, and is then qualified to direct the other (slave) through training and discipline with the intention to cause and assure obedience, which, as I have defined it, is an alignment of the will.

A slave cannot choose its Owner; that has been destined. An Owner cannot choose His slave because that, too, has been destined. We are either fulfilling our destiny or fulfilling our need to grow egotistically, but each is a different pursuit. Any time we're shopping, and comparison of wants and needs is brought up, we are picking a Master/slave partner. This should never be confused for Born slavery. Within that context, decide to obey The Owner, or decide to develop its slave résumé in order to negotiate its relationship with a Master. Either is legitimate. Just be clear which one you're doing.

slave 7:

SlaveMaster absolutely loves slaves. They are His passion and reason for existence, and He treats them with warmth, love and kindness as He helps them live to their fullest potential. After all, His slaves are a part of Himself.

Being Born slave

slave 7:

SlaveMaster and 7 often see in the world those with a fierce denial of life. For us, this is extreme. Those who call Born slavery extreme most often are other Masters and slaves. "Now, that's going too far!" says Ego. Usually, this judgment is based on a lack of understanding, or some kind of fear. For us, Born slavery is the most natural thing in the world.

Being SlaveMaster's Born slave means that the slave is His slave of Destiny. The slave has worked with SlaveMaster to the point that the slave has experienced sufficient loss of ego, such that the inner core of the slave person has come to life, unhampered and untainted by the human baggage that had covered it up. The slave can see and feel a whole Spirit Being within (or whatever you may choose to call it), that seems both brand-new and familiar. It is who the slave has always been. It is the true self revealed, just now freed from the layers and layers of stuff life on earth had heaped upon it. This does not mean that the ego has vanished forever, but rather just for a period, enough for the slave to experience its real self, to forever know and never again be denied, which then enables the slave to keep the ego at bay throughout life and live true to its slave nature.

"Birth" is a time of extreme clarity in which the slave may say, "Wow, who is that living inside me? i see you! What happened to 'me'?"   What i thought was me was really only a big nothing, only a superficial cover. And who is this inside me now? It's the real me! And the real me is this Slave Spirit thing that belongs to..." The slave knows it is Home with its Owner and that the Spirit is free to live as the slave it is. It feels like arrival, it feels like Birth, and it is amazing and joyous. This kind of "Birth" is not limited to slaves, but rather is a spiritual experience available to every human being: an awakening of the true self. For slaves, it just so happens that the true self turns out to be slave.

If we look at it from the standpoint of ego (or false self) vs. true self, then only the false self is the result of nurture, and the real self is the result of nature. Being Born as slave means the actualization of the real self, free of environmentally created ego needs and issues.

SlaveMaster often states that a strong, healthy and ready ego is needed before one can truly move into Born slavery and spiritual adulthood. This developed ego is strong enough to be destroyed, and the being inside taken low, where it is natural to go. Most slaves this slave has encountered over the years yearn to be LOW. Beautifully low. Where pretense ends. Low is as good as high. A refusal of the low is a limitation that will stop the completion of experiencing, and serving, the whole circle of existence. A refusal of the low is an act of saying no; it is a limitation and a disobedience. The Universe is in the completion of all things. We cannot choose to leave certain things out, or the circle will remain unfinished. So, should the low ever beckon, heed the call.

Born slavery is not a relationship to be negotiated between a Master and slave. Born slavery is a spiritual connection between an Owner and Born slave. Born slavery is about self-actualization. Entering slavery to SlaveMaster is more akin to entering a monastery than to entering a relationship.

SlaveMaster often states that a slave will not reach Birth if the slave is desiring and looking for Birth. It is when the slave authentically just doesn't give a damn anymore that things happen. Born slavery may appear extreme to anyone not designed for it, but for those of us who are, it is our comfort zone, our naturalness, and our lives. Trying to live in any other way would be extreme.

CONNECTION
An Article by SlaveMaster

None of us is prepared and qualified to exercise a free-will choice until we have fully developed egotistically. We need an almost arrogant confidence about our ability to achieve before we are ready to obey. When we are ready, free will can be exercised, either to choose to consciously give up free will, or to continue to pretend that we're acting from free will instead of all the influencing factors that cause us to behave as we do.

Nothing about spiritual evolution — going from spiritual childhood, to adolescence, and then onto adulthood — has anything to do with religion. Religion plays a critical part in each of our lives, but our spiritual lives are not defined by religion any more than they are defined by our work environment, our family or any other single influence. All of these experiences are how we develop.

Our drive to be happy is a search for being authentic, and finding and being who we are created to be. Who we are will always be about what we can do for the world, and not what we can do for us. The only reason to have any capacity is to influence the world according to the Universal plan.

What we think is control, viewed from the mature spiritual perspective, is nothing more than telling the Universe what we want to have happen. That's like telling the Creator how to do Its job. Consistent with that, ordinary prayer is about asking the Universe for Its help to achieve what we have already told IT we expect. Any desire that has to do with what we want is an egotistic desire and, therefore, has nothing to do with being obedient or "connected." So long as we are fulfilling goals we have identified and defined, we are only fulfilling selfish needs. When we no longer determine the goals we are pursuing, and instead are given the goals, then we are living obediently connected. I know that's not how it looks to any of us while we are still developing egotistically.

Connection is an alignment of wills. Obedience is the word used most often to describe the act of alignment of wills and is what creates the connection. After wills are aligned, there is only one will. When the "one" will is the Universe's will — the will of the intelligent "Source" — our own will must be ignored. There is no alignment so long as dual wills exist. So long as we still feel any right to our own will, there is no connection.

My personal alignment occurred through a series of events (that I wouldn't wish on My worst enemy) that forced Me, finally, to swear that I would never believe anything I'm not living, and to not live any way that I don't believe. With a high IQ and scientific educational background, it was easy for Me to theorize many things, and I did. I could argue any point of view I wanted, and always felt as if I was winning every argument. I learned that this exercise of the ego is what made My ego feel good, and feel strong. This was all nothing more than My personal egotistic development, and it was critical to My capacity to ultimately obey.

Being connected is having no such desire to feel egotistically good and strong. Being connected is not caring how I feel about what I am given to say, do or think. Being connected is about receiving continuous assignments, none of which are subject to My review nor My consideration. Being connected is about giving up the right to say "no."

Most of us spend our life wondering what to do. We struggle to find the internal voice that makes us sure of everything we decide and pursue. That struggle always will continue until we swear, in advance, to do and say anything we will be given to do.

Egotistically, we are trained to hear the options presented, analyze and consider whether or not it makes sense, is reasonable, and something we want to do, before we say yes or no. The problem is that the Universe has never wasted a command. Until IT knows we will do anything asked of us, it will not give any order. The Universe will not play egotistic games with us.

Anything we think is an order isn't, not until we have exercised an absolute vow to accomplish anything we are given. Until that commitment is convincingly offered, we are exercising our egotistic wishes, and still developing our spiritual adolescence. The ego takes credit for what we accomplish from such exercise of our wills, and the ego claims the result to be "in control."

The Universe isn't vindictive. So, it doesn't cause us to fail simply because we are making our decisions egotistically. We interpret the Universe's kind nature at letting us achieve what we want egotistically as being control. What it is, in fact, is how we are trained to have confidence. We are "connected" only when that confidence is given away in unqualified obedience.

Expressions of "free will" and being "connected" cannot occur simultaneously. Each is the diametric opposite of the other. Being connected is the result of having used free will to permanently surrender any right to free will. If free will is still an option, then we're not yet "connected" and that surrender has not occurred.

The Universe only fills out signed checks. Free will is the right to decide whether or not to sign each check. The Universe will not provide orders to anyone who still holds that right.

Like everyone, I presume, I tried to trick the Universe into thinking I was sworn to obey, while still holding the option to accept or reject any assignment given. The Universe, I learned, cannot be tricked. Either I obey or I don't. The Universe knows that until I have said "yes" before any order is given, I am not obeying at all. The right to consider the options is disobedience. Once the options are considered, when we proceed, we are merely only agreeing, and not obeying. The Universe will not give options for us to consider agreeing with. It's "all or none." We obey or we don't. It's that simple and that demanding.

I thought I was smart. Since I could out-argue everyone else, I thought I could trick the Universe as well with the same "smart" twists in logic and conclusions. It works something like this: Someone offers Me an orange. I respond "No, thank you." From that, the one offering the orange concludes that I have decided to starve Myself to death, and then proclaims that I am clearly "wrong" because having a death wish makes no sense. When, in fact, I had just eaten and only refused the orange because I was not hungry. Using this technique, no one could disagree with anyone or any concept. It's a technique I've used and seen everyone in egotistic development use. It's a part of growing up spiritually.

Every time I used this technique, either with others or with the Universe, I arrogantly felt I had won the argument. From that I assumed everyone could see how smart and how "right" I was. After all, a death wish is not a good thing, and I knew I could get everyone to agree with that. I felt so smart and so smug. However, everyone could see right through My logic, but knew how important winning was to Me, so I wasn't confronted. That made it easy to feel as though I continued to win.

The Universe doesn't play word games. The Universe gave Me the exact life I needed to understand that I had no control over anything, and that trying to control was telling "God" what to do, and that the ordinary prayer of asking for things was simply a confirmation of My arrogance from telling the Creator what I expected of IT.

Being connected is having no religion to broker My relationship with the Source. Being connected is having no sense of self other than being an instrument for the Universal plan. Being connected is knowing there is no reason to have talent or skill unless it is to support the Universal plan which will never be shared with Me. Being connected is accepting that the most I can ever know is what I am personally supposed to do in each moment.

When connected, the responsibility is only to the "order." It is not My business to even know the results of what I do, nor to take any credit for what is accomplished through Me. I cannot be connected and view any capacity or influence that I have as any more than a gift. Each gift is either from My parents, My peers, My family, My teachers, My religious influence, or the gift of My orders from the Universe. To take credit, and to claim free will, is blatant arrogance and disrespect of the Creator and of Its control. I learned how impossible it is to claim to have both free will and to be spiritual.

Spirituality begins when we surrender free will. Until then, I, like everyone else, thought I was spiritual because I didn't deny the existence of some unseen intelligence that existed outside Myself. Admitting to the existence didn't make Me spiritual. Obeying made Me spiritual. Admitting to the existence of a spiritual intelligence merely kept My options open.

Only the ego is arrogant enough to try to accomplish being connected, to gain the benefits, and then turn around and try to take claim and credit for those benefits. The only claim I can make is to the quality and consistency of My obedience. Everything else IS a gift, purely, clearly and completely.

An absolute freedom from what others think comes from being connected. Having others disagree with My experiences is, at most, an amusement that comes from remembering being devoid of My connection and so sure of My erroneous egotistic views back then. The same freedom from taking credit for what I do is a freedom from criticism. None of My actions or words is Me, and none of it is Mine. Try to claim it, and the Universe will stop giving the commands that allow IT to accomplish Its tasks through Me. The Universe cannot be misled into believing I obey when I don't just so I can get orders which I could then abuse. We cannot abuse the privilege of being given orders, the privilege of being connected. The orders will stop.

What I do as an Owner, then, is act from the commands I am given. Because none of My intention comes from Me, all the S/M experiences and all the decisions I make regarding My slaves are consistent with all their life experiences. Those experiences give evidence to a slave that My commands could not be egotistically based. What each slave had to initially take on "faith" becomes a knowing. The doubt and the need to question disappear.

The slave learns and inherits the Owner's connection. Knowing The Owner's connection allows a slave the same opportunity to live by obedience, and to surrender the ego and an egotistic agenda and limitations. Like being pregnant, there is no such thing as being partly obedient. We either are or we aren't. So long as we claim free will, we aren't.

Because the Universe doesn't give a connection without the deepest commitment we are capable of (that we will always and only obey), there is no "sometimes on" and "sometimes off." The unwavering consistency is what gives the feeling of being home, and the freedom to relinquish doubt.

Any discussion that continues to honor the value and legitimacy of the ego and its free will precludes the admission and discussion of living spiritually. One is a means to the other, but they don't co-exist. Arguments that revolve around free will and egotistic agendas that make us proud, powerful, or capable of intimidating others are not discussions of finding and accepting our spiritual lives. Instead, they are discussions of how we prepare for our spiritual lives.

Having said that, accepting our spiritual lives IS spiritual adulthood. Not everyone is yet ready to enter adulthood. Adulthood is possible only after completing our spiritual childhood and adolescence. The process isn't linear enough to say there are those ahead of and behind us in the process, but we each can use help along the way. What's important to remember is that someone who isn't where we are right now isn't "wrong," but simply at a different place in their development. Respecting that allows us each to learn the most from each other.

Being spiritual — being connected — requires giving our entire lives to our unwavering obedience. No part of our selves, or our lives, can be excluded. The difficulty isn't in qualifying to become connected. The challenge is in letting go of our limited, egotistic, free-willed and self-controlled lives. Graduating from spiritual adolescence requires so much ego that we become reluctant to hand over what we have worked so hard to achieve. However, when ready, handing it over is all we have to do.

This is what happiness is.

slave 7:

Life, this slave concludes, is, at some point, all about connection. We live, we struggle, we agonize, we find our safe places, we wait . . . until we are ready . . . and the Universe is ready for us . . . to connect.

Being Different

slave 7:

This slave understands slave-fear very, very well. This slave, as it is and does now, would have scared the shit out of itself some years ago. This slave also understands slave-misery very, very well. it lived with it for years on end: that desperate loneliness, that feeling of being freakishly different, that feeling of "I must be insane." And the fear of self, and of some crazy Master. But life carries us on. And we can and do reach a place of peace and understanding. But we get there when we get there. When we are meant to get there.

Being Machine

SlaveMaster:

It is interesting to see being a machine associated with that machine not being a gift, and having no capacity to love or be loved. In other writings you have learned that while a machine, I am convinced that slaves are this world's greatest resource. Being able to turn them off and on doesn't diminish that fact, but, instead, enhances it. Machines have superior ability to accomplish and are undistracted and undiminished by egotistic, selfish agenda. That's why slaves are unequalled in life.

Celebrate where you are. Learn everything you can about your current state. Leave no leaf unturned in understanding yourself. Live, however, with the knowledge that with the potential of being the finest existence alive — a machine made of flesh and blood— that a life that can't even be dreamed right now is not only possible but probable given how you feel, who you are, and the potential for greatness that is intrinsic in all authentic slaves.

I could argue that human beings don't walk. For the first part of their lives that is true. At any given moment on earth there are millions of human beings that don't have the capacity to walk. There is an error, however, in believing that just because millions can't walk, that humans are not designed to walk. Because slavery doesn't feel like being a machine, it doesn't mean that finding the blissful machine state, operated by another who lives inside it, isn't achievable.

slave 7:

This slave can say that the first time SlaveMaster called this slave a machine was a very troubling experience. This slave felt all the negative connotations of the word "machine" when applied to a living creature. It took only a few minutes of talk, however, to understand what He meant by "machine" and to know that He did not mean to suggest that His slave is nothing but a collection of cold, lifeless, disposable parts. That is only what this slave's ego thinks a machine is.

SlaveMaster is in love with technology and machines. He sees machines as the highest, purest art form humanity can attain. Don't show Him the Mona Lisa, show Him a well-oiled, well-designed machine. SlaveMaster sees great art and spirit in functionality and design and in their actualization in a product we call a machine. What others often interpret as cold and distant and as disrespectful to the slave, we experience as the highest form of intimacy, love, freedom and esteem.

A slave, in SlaveMaster language, is a machine because it operates for the Universe purely, obediently, and as the highest realization of form and function the Universe attains in humanity. So, if SlaveMaster ever calls you a machine, please say "thank you," because He has just paid you the highest compliment He knows how.

Being One with Master

slave 7:

The body is an actual machine, but there is a soul inside that machine. That soul is NOT the slave's soul, however. The soul is that of the slave's Owner. This is the distinction SlaveMaster makes between being a "Master and slave" versus being "Owner and slave." As He uses the terms, Owner and slave share the same soul; Master and slave do not.

This might be why you have the fetish desire to be slave: the soul inside the machine yearns to be home with the main part of itself, and that main part only exists in and through the slave's true Owner.

Once a slave accepts that it belongs to a Master/Owner, it just follows the orders. A slave doesn't pick and choose what to obey and what not to obey, nor does it consider any selfish desires. And, amazingly, it all works. The right Owner with the right slave can just meld, and the slave's only desire becomes to be at One with the Master/Owner. If a slave hesitates to obey an order, the key is to know where that hesitation is coming from — the ego

57

or the slave heart. If it is coming from the heart (or spirit), then there may be a real problem with the slave's connection to the Master/Owner.

Permission is not a word SlaveMaster uses in regard to slaves. Permission implies that the slave is a separate individual and wants something that the Owner then has to allow for. SlaveMaster's slaves have no wants, except to be at One with the Owner. To be at One with the Owner is to have only His will and no other. We are talking total obedience here, right down to the slave only wanting what He wants, but with the right connection, it is natural and easy. It is not about doing what somebody else wants. It is about accepting that what you want is coming from another, and is not your own. As SlaveMaster says, we do not own our soul; the soul owns us. It is about obeying the motivations one naturally feels.

slave 7 feels connected to its Owner as One, and real evidence of this arises from time to time as SlaveMaster and this slave subtly—and sometimes not so subtly — "read each other's minds" or are completely in sync. 7 knows that it can know its Owner's Will without any words being spoken; 7 knows His will as its own. 7 knows that its life has improved and has never been better, and that it continues to improve the more deeply and consistently it lives true to its "truest and deepest" slave nature within. 7 knows that life makes a lot more sense to it now that it is slave and that pieces of the puzzle of its life have fallen neatly into place as its "truest and deepest" nature is more and more fully allowed to live. 7 knows that slavery to SlaveMaster is beautiful and healthy, a great gift that it cherishes. 7 knows that it doesn't need to know any more than what it already knows.

SlaveMaster often writes that His slaves are an extension of himself and not pieces of property. SlaveMaster does not see His slaves as property nor as voluntary servants. His slaves are literally His own body parts.

This slave used to so desperately long for connection to a Man in slavery. It found a few good Men over the years, but despite its deep yearnings for slavery, this slave felt an overwhelming stress and urge to run from these Men. They didn't feel like Home, this slave now realizes. When this slave met SlaveMaster, it found Home.

If all the Universe is a jigsaw puzzle and we are all pieces designed to fit exactly into only one place, then the Born slave fits exactly into the piece that is its Owner, and nowhere else. And this is Home. This is the slave's connection to the Cosmos, to all the Universe, to all Creation. So, when this slave hears of slaves who tend to beat themselves up for not sticking with a particular Master or for not being absolutely obedient to that Master, this slave suspects that perhaps the slave simply hasn't found Home. Or, at least, the slave hasn't yet found the sense of Home in that Master/Owner. Being Obedient is easy when one truly feels at Home.

SlaveMaster values and holds His slaves so dear that He knows them as a part of His own body, which he feels as warm and intimate and right. His slaves accept His leadership so strongly, and embrace Obedience to such a degree, His slaves are "connected" to Him. And, indeed, we believe that spiritually we are absolutely connected.

The desire to be dependent is the desire to be linked, to be connected. It is a call to intimacy.

Being Owned

SlaveMaster:

A slave looking for its Owner is entering into a contract that demands only "obey every order." An Owner's contract is: "Act in the best interest of the slave." That is the totality of the Divine contract which binds an Owner to His destined slave.

When either the Master or the potential slave starts modifying that contact with "Must look like . . ." or "Must provide the service of . . ." it is NOT an Ownership, as I define the term, but a Master/slave relationship that is under discussion and consideration.

Once it is clear that a Master/slave arrangement is being put together, the slave is expected, by necessity, to protect itself and maintain self-responsibility, and anyone who describes his or her own needs is not offering Ownership. A slave is either ready to obey, or still needs to prepare for Ownership by shopping for and negotiating with a Master. Some are never meant to be a destined slave, and a negotiated relationship might be the ultimate position.

If an Owner can't exclusively give Love and Power, that person isn't qualified to be an Owner, but is, instead, in the process of their own development. We can't give what we don't have. Until we know how to offer something without any expectation of return, we don't know how to love. Until we feel powerful, without pretending or posturing to do so, we can't give any power away. The Owner must grow into being qualified to give the slave growth. It isn't in the technique. Everything is in the intention and what we are willing to do to be qualified to hold that intention. Fools and poseurs can hurt, break, abuse, punish, humiliate and harm another. Prisons are full of such people who are successful at doing so. The challenge and satisfaction for a Born slave's Owner comes from becoming so pure that the unblemished gift of Love and Power can be given without any expectation of reward or return. If there is any expectation, then it isn't a gift, but only an exchange.

slave 7:

When actually considering a Master for real-time slavery, 7 asked itself the following kinds of questions: Why does this Master deserve to own me? What qualifies this Master to Master anybody, especially me? How can this Master IMPROVE and EMPOWER the quality of my life? Am i only desperate and turned on, or is there a real connection here? How will i be a happier and better person as a result of being His slave?

In short, all slaves are different, and any Master worthy of Ownership will be able to sense, develop and use that uniqueness, as opposed to prescribing too extensively in advance. Further, all slaves need to be developed in different ways, so shackling, for example, may work for some slaves and not others. Again, each slave is unique and has unique needs for the journey into full slavery. And the right Master for you knows that.

Being True To Self

slave 7:

SlaveMaster says that while growing up and finding Himself, being a SlaveMaster would have never been the job He would have chosen. He simply found His natural life. SlaveMaster says: "We get the life we are given, and the one we are designed for, not the one we want."

Birth of slave

SlaveMaster:

7 has reached a benchmark of Birth, and that brings with it a certain set of experiences and knowing. All the rest of us have a different set.

Coming Out

slave 7:

This slave supposes coming out as slave or Master is not much different than coming out as LGBQT over the past decades. It would seem that motivation and intent are the real issues. Is the intent to hide? Is the intent to inform so that an open and strengthened familial bond may be present? Is the need to simply be one's self, to allow one's self to flourish openly? Whatever the case, our connection to others is limited by an inability to be ourselves with them and to communicate fully with them. Sometimes the limit will remain in others, and maybe that is how it should be. Maybe we are meant to separate from family and not artificially hold on. Integrity, or living as authentically and openly as possible, builds what needs to be built, gives what needs to be given, and destroys what needs to be destroyed.

Confidence

slave 7:

This slave sees slaves who struggle and struggle with life, and resist and resist slavery, though they can't seem to stop contacting SlaveMaster for "advice" once in a while, over stretches of 10 years and more. They are distraught, but they can't turn to slavery because it is too extreme. They look for answers in psychology, in self-help books, in philosophies, in this guru or that, in this expert or that... anything to get out of following through with the desire they can't get rid of. This slave doesn't diminish the value of looking in all these directions. In fact, that is exactly what it did for 20+ years before finding SlaveMaster. But when all alternatives are exhausted, it is the strength within that will give the support and lead the right way, no matter how extreme it may seem.

Connection

SlaveMaster:

My confidence in the orders I give, and a slave's trust in me, comes from recognizing that all internal orders My slave receives directly match the external orders the slaves receives from me.

The slave realizing the order within confirms the validity of the Master-slave connection and demonstrates the validity of My obedience, as I can see the oneness of Will in both Myself and My slave. Ultimately, it is this reality that replaces faith with knowing a slave is with its destined owner.

In other words, anyone can issue a verbal order, and anyone willing can follow it. But if the Master and slave can confirm that they are acting upon an internal voice that is stating the same thing, this demonstrates a connection between them, as they are experiencing a Oneness of will. SlaveMaster can confirm His own sense of what the natural order is (i.e., His own obedience) when He sees that His slave is following the order without Him ever verbalizing it. When we have such explicit evidence, we come to know, rather than have faith, that the connection is real.

A Poem by slave 7:

Connection is a state of being
In which one is aware that over time
One's obedience is true and effective
In the world and the
Lives of Others.

Connection is a state of being
In which one is aware
That one's life lies on a path
And that when one stays on that path

One may receive in ways
Not directly and not immediately
Related to one's giving

Connection is a state of being
In which one is aware
That one's personal history
Was planned in order to create
One that works well in the
Destiny the Universe has laid out

Connection is a state of being
In which one gives freely into the void
Of not caring about a return
Nor about another's reactions,
Feelings or state of connectedness
In any given moment.

Consciousness

slave 7:

What exactly is the slave consciousness? That is not easy to answer. There certainly is a consciousness present, and it can decide to not live as slave and go through life without the Owner. But, as most of you must know, that feels awful. Or, at the very least, it creates a sense of something missing in life, a yearning. The slave soul wants and needs to go "home." That is, it needs to join with the Owner soul. And the only way to reunite with the Owner soul is to live in spiritual obedience. That is the glue, the connector, the container that holds it all together.

And what does the slave consciousness within His machine get out of this? Bliss, happiness and the sense that it is doing the right thing with its life.

Control

SlaveMaster:

What we believe is intended to change through time. The change can occur during a single flogging, through months of a relationship or by having our lives fall apart to show us we never did have any control in the first place, which is a lesson we must all learn eventually.

Desperation

slave 7:

It would seem that proceeding with a Master out of desperation is unwise, dangerous, and untrue to the spirit. Desperate desire for a Master can cause a slave to act out of selfish want rather than authentic need. It blocks the slave's good sense and power of judgment.

Desperation creates disobedience. In fact, it is this slave's experience (this slave understands this only in retrospect) that desperation is the feeling that arises when the slave, desperately in search of a Master, is about to take a misstep due to the desire for self-satisfaction, rather than truly stepping ahead to the right Master.

Desperate desire can be understood as an Order to not proceed— a wall that one should not climb over, a barrier that one should respect — a red flag. It creates a set of demands from the desperate slave that must be lived up to, which is exactly the wrong place at which to begin one's slavery. Desperation can cause one to settle for less than Right.

WHAT IS A SLAVE'S DESTINY?
An Article by SlaveMaster

A Born slave's life is spiritual, and there is no way to understand slavery without generally understanding how life works. The spiritual world is the real world, and every slave must discover that before fully becoming slave.

It is the Owner and Operator of the spiritual world that grants slavery. It is that force, intelligence, and order that I generally refer to as "Universe" that declares when someone is finally qualified to be a slave. What name IT has won't make a difference. Just as what we believe doesn't change the truth, what we call something doesn't change its nature or purpose.

Every man or woman of destiny has two phases in his or her life, separated by a defining moment. During the first phase, we learn, develop and grow into feeling personally successful. During the second phase, we live the personally unique destined life that was realized and confirmed during the defining moment. There is only one destiny per person, and no two of us can have the same destiny.

The second phase will always be what the Universe intends it to be. There will be no way to predict it, and no way to influence it. If what we're doing is predictable, then it isn't destined. What has happened before cannot be a part of destiny. Once a path is taken, it can never be repeated, no matter how valuable or worthy the path. That's the nature of destiny.

During the first phase of a slave's life, the challenge is first to feel personal value and independent success. Second, he must discover and confirm he was created to be a slave. Third, a slave must determine that he personally possesses the motivation and commitment to the process required to become the slave he was created to be. A slave has to know what he's willing to give, and give up, for the acquisition of his destiny.

The final defining step is different for a slave. It is the only distinguishing difference between a slave and any other person in pursuit of destiny. Who a slave is was given to another by his Creator. Therefore, the slave needs to find that man or woman who carries the slave's purpose.

There must be no value judgment assigned to being destined to be a slave. Despite the egotistic training we receive to be independent, self-directed, and free of co-dependency at all costs, slavery is a legitimate destiny. Ego training is a legitimate requirement of phase one, to enable our egotistic success. It is not a part of anyone's destiny. Slaves are creatures different from humans, but not lesser than humans.

Being a slave puts a man or woman into a position to accomplish greater tasks with less effort, because of the shared nature of his or her life, and provides a route to accomplishing the defining moment at a more rapid pace. A slave is only part of another. A division of labor to succeed is created because there is more than one part. A slave is made of obedience, and finds his or her only pleasure to be the accomplishment of a lifelong stream of orders that directs all of life's activities.

There is a reason certain men and women have been selected to be slave. We can never know the reason, but we can be sure that it is because the Universe has work it wants accomplished that only a slave can accomplish. Others, with other destinies, are intended to do the work they can uniquely do. Slaves are designed to accomplish the impossible and the improbable because they are designed to obey. They are uniquely qualified to accomplish that which they are designed to accomplish. No one else can complete a slave's task in life.

Being slave is a very high calling. It is nothing to be ashamed of or to feel lesser about. Just the opposite, being slave is to possess a nature that is superior to characteristics which we humans exhibit. Slaves don't have inhibitions and limitations. Slaves are not capable of dishonesty or deceit. Slaves can have no agenda of their own, which leaves them pure and capable only of totally unselfish lives. They are suitable for the acceptance of unlimited trust.

Destiny also makes it equally the Owner's task to find the other parts of himself. Only a destined Owner can develop the raw materials presented to him by a potential slave into a powerful man or woman of destiny. Each Owner will have many parts He has to find. Each slave will have his one Owner to find. Many others help a slave along the way, but only one person is destined to carry a slave's purpose. The Universe didn't spread a slave's purpose around the countryside to make it available for anyone who wanted to pick it up and give it to the intended slave. A slave's purpose is as precisely assigned as the slavery itself. It is the complementary part of the same destiny.

Destiny is precise. For those who want to achieve it, everything must be done as it was intended to be. Egotistic-determined goals are the antithesis of our destiny. We either do the Universe's work or we do our own. We can't do both.

Every slave is led, or banged around, through life to develop his value, and to show him that his life won't be complete without his Owner. No matter what a slave does, his purpose is still missing until he finds his Owner. Most of life's experience is intended to prove to the slave what won't work. Finally, when the slave is ready, the Universe provides the opportunity to know and accept his Owner — his destiny — and the process which will develop the raw material the slave offers to his Owner. It's all the same decision.

The slave provides willingness, honesty and the raw material. Only the Owner can bend, temper, weld, hammer and shape the raw material into a beautiful and respected tool, like the way a sword is built. Then, just like the sword, the sword is known by its Owner and the strength of the sword is the sword's ability to obey and be used as the Owner intends it. If the sword bends whenever the sword feels like it, the sword is useless. A sword with its own agenda is worthless.

It is the Owner's job to recognize the raw material, and to direct the use of the tool as the Creator intends it to be used. The sword fulfills the Owner's needs and purpose, and in being used, the sword becomes a critical part of the Owner's need, purpose and process. The Owner cannot do what he was created to do without the sword, and the sword has no purpose without the Owner. If the sword reserves the right to make decisions on its own, then it can't help the Owner with his purpose.

A sword without the Owner's purpose has no purpose. A sword isn't given, nor does it need, a purpose of its own. Nevertheless, it can still go down revered through history because of the results of its existence and use.

Likewise, a slave has no separate purpose. The slave has NO purpose except to obey, and has no responsibility except to obey, and has no right except to obey. The last thing that a slave would ever want to know is how he personally feels about any order. While he egotistically examines the last order, he misses the next one and risks influencing the order.

It is the single loyalty to obedience, the embracing of each order, which sets the slave free. Because a slave obeys, he can feel the spirit that the Owner has built and empowered inside, a spirit which is the Owner's spirit. The slave becomes light, joyous, spontaneous, creative, intuitive and inspired. The slave can do no wrong because all of his negative intention has been replaced with obedience.

The obedience also protects the slave. The slave can risk being spontaneous and natural only because the slave KNOWS he will obey, and knows he has an Owner who will issue any order needed to protect him. The order is of no value without the obedience.

Once completely free to only obey, the slave can feel the Owner's purpose inside. The slave development process teaches a slave that the spirit the Owner builds inside the slave is the same spirit as the Owner's, and he learns that when the Owner's spirit is directed, so is the slave's. The slave begins to feel direction through the Owner's spirit directly, from inside, and knows the Owner has the same direction. Because the Owner obeys, the slave can obey, and does.

The Owner doesn't get one order and the slave a different one. There can be no conflict. The slave knows that the orders the slave feels inside are the same as those given to his Owner. Since there is only one order, there is no conflict. The Owner's job is to both give orders directly and to enforce those orders that are given to the Owner's spirit inside the slave. This prevents the slave from making excuses for not doing what his Creator, the Universe, gives the slave to do.

The Owner doesn't have to personally issue every order. Once the slave recognizes that his mind, body and spirit ARE the Owner, not as his property but as Himself, the slave acts, thinks, loves, and lives for the Owner, and only for the Owner, because that's all there is. There is no separate, distinct person that is slave. There is no one to have a second opinion. There is only the Owner's opinion and the Owner's opinion. There is only the Owner's will and the Owner's will. Slave development is the experience of this as true and real.

The slave development process leaves a slave with absolute moral certainty. In every moment, in every circumstance, the slave knows what to do. When the Owner is physically present, the slave accepts his orders directly. When the Owner is physically apart, the slave obeys the Owner's spirit inside with the same passion and dedication as he obeys the orders which come from the Owner's mouth.

It is the existence of the Owner's spirit internally that convinces the slave that he is slave. No one can make up a spirit for someone else to feel, to live by and to be. No amount of punishment and brain-washing could ever create a part of another man's soul for someone who looks distinct from his Owner, but is actually ONLY a part of his Owner. The soul, the spirit, can't be invented by man.

Since a slave lives only in the Owner's soul, he can spend his whole life doing what feels like play, whether making multi-million dollar corporate decisions, deciding which streets to use to drive home, or whom to love. When a man obeys, and has an Owner, and has sworn unqualified obedience to that Owner, everything he does is the right thing. Every action is directed by the Universe, and to accomplish the Universe's purpose. When a man obeys, the consequence of the action is none of his business. What is done honestly, from a place of power given by the Owner, and from a place of love given by the Owner, is always the right thing to do.

The only pleasure a slave can feel is to fulfill an order, to obey. When in constant obedience without the right or desire to do anything else, everything a slave does is pleasure, and, everything the slave does is morally correct. A slave cannot perform an immoral act, an angry act, a dishonest act, a deceitful act, a vengeful act, a spiteful act, or any negative act, because he obeys instead.

The Owner is morally responsible for everything a slave does for the rest of his life, after Birth. There is only one soul among the Owner and His slaves, and what happens with one will happen with all.

Birth is when destiny begins, when a slave does only what his Creator wants him to do and nothing more, and nothing less. Destiny begins when a slave accepts that he isn't himself, but is only a part of another, when a man knows that he can only obey and that nothing else is his business, forever. It is a moment when spirituality is experienced first- hand, and the personal attention of the Universe becomes known. It is a final goodbye to life directed by the ego and any claim to a self that is separate from the Owner.

A SlaveMaster is an Owner. A Master is not an Owner. Masters can come and go. There could be several through a lifetime. There can only be one Owner, and it has to be the right one, because an Owner is who the Universe gave a slave's soul to when the slave was created. Masters have a critical role in a slave's life, but the purpose isn't to own. It is potentially possible that someone could be both a slave's SlaveMaster and Master, but it is not necessarily the case because of the vast difference in purpose.

Through life a slave can feel the soul he is meant to be, but can never fully inherit it until he accepts his slavery. Slave development is a process that concludes in a single moment in which the Universe who created the slave gives a slave his intended destiny. Slavery can't be given by the Owner, it can only be given by the Creator. That keeps the Owner in line, and in obedience! Otherwise, the Owner could play favorites and make mistakes. He could hand out slavery as a reward. The Universe is far too wise to allow that to happen.

Slavery has to be given EXACTLY as the Universe wants it given. It doesn't make any difference how anyone, including the Owner or the slave, feels about any part of the protocol or process required to produce it. There is nothing to negotiate, nothing to bargain or contract for. It must be precisely as it must be, or it will never be at all.

This — ALL — is the minimum requirement to be a slave. This isn't something that might happen someday for some slave. Any man or woman who hasn't achieved what I have described here might know that they are meant to be slave, but are not slave yet. Slavery is not a decision. It is a gift from the Universe in acknowledgment of having become one of the Universe's soldiers. When I witness that event, is when the tattoo of achievement and the Birth sequence number is assigned to a man, not one second before.

Until the above is accepted as true, there can be no understanding of authentic slavery. So long as there is any implication that an Owner, the SlaveMaster, and his slave are two men, there is no way to grasp the meaning of slavery. The word "slave" has been misused in alternate contexts, and for alternative reasons, but it isn't what slavery is, or was ever meant to be. It isn't my job to change how a word is used. Anyone can use any word they want at any time. Slavery is what slavery is, and what word is used, or how it is used, won't change any part of it.

Slaves who have not found their slavery are men or women who are still forced to live as though they are separate. It is like having a script in a play that won't end. There is no way to exit the stage and go to "real life" for those created to be slave, but not developed and Born.

This is the source of the frustration, the extreme measures slaves go to, the feelings of depression and despair that they're commonly faced with. It is why a slave justifies and feels that it's okay to abandon everything, against the slave's common sense, for someone who will treat him like a slave, only to find that he still isn't fulfilled. When the true nature of slavery is understood, it is easy to see where the one-handed fiction has come from, and why the feelings that slaves have are being experienced. They know inside they can have no limits. They simply don't yet understand the framework in which it must happen.

Until a slave is a part of another, he or she doesn't know who they are at all. They can have a lot of success, and play at being slave in a lot of relationships, but they still don't know who they are. Because slaves have to be talented and creative to perform the jobs their creator intends for them, they are good at acting like they have found who they are. They are very good actors and play their scripts well. An Owner knows when it's acting, and sees a precious part of himself in the slave he looks at. An Owner doesn't even notice the image, the facade, that's been created, because it is of no importance to Him.

As a guess as to why part of our species have been created and are destined to become a slave, some theorize that the resurgence of authentic slavery has to do with preparing for the new Millennium and the Age of Aquarius. Others postulate other theories. Why doesn't matter. That slavery is becoming important, critical and respected as an existence is observable. I expect it won't be long before there will be awe and respect in people when they learn that someone is a slave.

I also predict that slaves will be expected to be the models of how to live in the new Millennium, and that might be the least of their tasks, through obedience, for and as the Owner who has built them and cares enough to issue the orders.

If a man feels fulfilled while "living the script," he isn't slave at all, even if he uses the name "slave." People have the capacity to live like a dog, like furniture, or like a slave, and that doesn't a dog, furniture, or a slave make.

Without Birth, a slave is still acting human. So long as a slave acts human, or pretends to be his own individual self, he is only acting. Any question or process which leaves the slave as a separate individual, capable of disobedience and of making decisions about who he is, whether they are better decisions or not, is still being human, not slave.

The rules that apply to humans do not apply to slaves, and the rules that apply to slaves don't apply to humans. To treat a human like a slave is to abuse him. To treat a slave like a human is to abuse the slave. They are different creatures, with different requirements and different needs.

If someone expresses something about what is good for a human, it probably is not good for a slave. People with a psychology background are normally the worst of all at understanding slavery because of their need to see slaves as human. Psychologists find it discomforting and disorienting to not be able to pigeon-hole into human behavior slots how a slave behaves and must be treated.

Slaves are given orders; everything else for a slave is abuse. Slaves are better than human, they have a higher calling, and have more to accomplish with their life than most humans. They are men and women of destiny, which few humans achieve. To be destined is the minimum requirement for a slave, not the best they can hope for.

What is stated here is a lot to accept. That's why it takes time to become a slave. I don't have a choice about being an Owner and giving men their slavery, and slaves don't have a choice about being slave.

Not only is what I have stated a lot to accept, a slave must personally experience every part of it to be true. Nothing can be taken on my word or anyone else's. It all has to be individually experienced and confirmed to accept the demands and freedom of slavery. That's another reason why it takes time, why slave development is a lengthy process.

Some have suggested to me that they could become slave in a weekend. It's not going to happen any more than you could become a doctor in a weekend, no matter how true the calling, no matter how motivated, no matter how prepared for the challenge.

I hope these thoughts will help you get a better grip on this. I know how challenging it is to believe. It took decades for me to accept it. I have experienced it all to be true, over and over, but I'm still in no better position to defend nor better explain why than anyone else. I don't have to understand physics to know the sun will come up every day, and I don't know why the Universe has selected certain men and women to be slave. But it has, and they have an ominous task to perform that would look impossible if they weren't slave, and living in obedience.

Additional Thoughts on Destiny:
SlaveMaster:

Life is what leads us to our slavery. Life isn't what gets in the way of our slavery. All of us here are pursuing slavery, or Mastery/Ownership as a destiny: None of us are prepared for our destiny until we actually are prepared for our destiny. In other words, we are not ready till we're ready. It is impossible to egotistically declare we want our slavery, Mastery or Ownership, and then magically get what we've declared we want. At best, our declaration of want is a prayer which puts our lives onto a path that prepares us for what we seek.

Hold constant thoughts about what we don't have and the Universe will hear that constant declaration as a prayer and put everything IT can in our lives to see that it remains as we see it and expect it to be. That's how our thoughts, prayers and lives work. Wanting blocks what we could have, and always delays what we need.

Accept where we are right now, with the present opportunities in front of us, do what obedience would dictate we should do, and we will move one step closer to fulfilling our Created design — our destiny.

Our current lesson could be one of forgiveness, honesty, integrity, love, vindictiveness, justice, fairness, spite or the biggest lesson of all, that none of us has any control over our lives. We make choices that coincidentally agree with the Divine plan, and we take egotistic credit for the outcome, which makes the lesson even harder to learn because we interpret what happens as evidence that we were right about our having control.

What we do in our lives is all about what we can do for everyone else. The only reason we improve personally is to get better and more efficient at serving the rest of the world as we were designed to according to our destiny. Forget that, make life about us and what we can get from it, how it can all be made better for us, and we're not in support of the Universal plan, and are therefore without Universal support in our activities. Then we claim frustration and cry about our disappointment.

The spiritual world is real. Our misconceptions about the nature of the spiritual world, or our lack of real acceptance of the reality of it, absolutely prevent the inheritance of our destinies. Until we only obey, until we accept the present as a gift, until we know life is not about us, until we embrace what we're given instead of always looking for what we don't have, we won't find our destiny.

Life moves in phases. First we must become tribal, learning and accepting the group values and in exchange being protected by the tribe. Second we must become egotistically strong to know that we have capacity, ability, worth, and are a resource. Third, destiny begins when we surrender who and what we are egotistically to the Divine purpose for which we were created.

Mastery, Ownership and slavery are not the usual destinies. It is a valuable gift and asset to have someone point out to us where we should go next in life, answer our questions while we do so, and help us maintain perspective to maximize the benefit we get from each lesson. It would be a dream fulfilled to see us become a community dedicated to mutual support and development of each other in the pursuit of our unique destinies.

When we find and accept our destiny, every other destiny is no longer an option. Once our personal destiny is identified, all hope of any other is gone. To develop enough egotistically, we have needed to become confident about our ability to do anything we put our minds to. Destiny takes all choice of what and who we'll be out of our hands.

Much of the development and evolution that prepares us for our destiny is in building the confidence and courage necessary to accept what life wants of us, forever abandoning what we want of life. Master, Owner and slave are who we are, not what we do, not how we do it nor how we want things done. It is much more than how we play or what role we'll take when we play. Finding reasons not to pursue our destiny is easy. The challenge is to find the reason and motivation to pursue our destiny.

slave 7:

SlaveMaster states that just as we do not suddenly volunteer during our teen years to be male or female, gay or straight, or of any particular race or body type, we do not volunteer to be slave. We simply are, since biological Birth, made to be slave, and we can't live satisfactorily or happily in any other way. We MUST join with the Being that we are a part of. That is what SlaveMaster means by saying that slavery is a Destiny. We have no choice. We simply are slave. Not a distinct individual owned as property, but literally the extra hands, feet, mind, mouth, etc. of our Owner Spirit.

DEVELOPMENT OF SLAVE
An Article by SlaveMaster

After you have done all the soul-searching, asked all the questions, and satisfied yourself that you have always been slave, you finally decide that you are ready to accept slavery as your destiny and are ready to begin your development. What happens then?

The decision has to have been made after you have determined that you are fully egotistically developed. You must know that you can be financially independent and can support yourself without anyone else's help. You have to have experience putting together successful relationships. You need to know that you can maintain your relationships with and responsibilities to your genetic family. You have to be in the best health that you can be, and know that you can maintain your health. You have to have control of your life, your profession, and your social needs and be able to maintain healthy friendships. Until you have it all, you don't have it to give away.

No one is ready to develop their destiny until they know they are individually capable of taking care of everything but their spiritual completion. Spiritually, a man preparing to accept his destiny has to be able to understand the spiritual world. There isn't any destiny to accept if you don't have a belief in a spiritual life, and have some understanding of how that might work. Destiny is a spiritual path. If there is no spiritual world, then there is no destiny. If there is no destiny, then Born slavery can't exist, because it is a form of destiny.

- **NOW YOU'RE READY TO BEGIN. WHAT DOES THAT MEAN?**

It means that you have committed yourself to obedience. Out of strength, not weakness, you have made a decision to accept the reality of your slavery. You are ready to be ordered into the circumstances and resulting experiences that will force you to fully prepare for your destiny.

It means that you have decided that you won't be able to anticipate the way your development will work. You understand that there is no development when you can anticipate what will happen. You want to be strengthened by the truth, and learn what it is like to live fully as a part of another. You understand the implications of "unqualified obedience."

There are several conditions that have to have been accepted to develop as a slave:

- **YOU MUST HAVE THE RIGHT TO END YOUR DEVELOPMENT.**

A slave can't burn any bridges to start his slave development. Burned bridges remove options from a slave's life. The challenge of becoming slave is one of finding, then learning through experience, that you have found and are pursuing the best possible life options. Destroying other options undermine, and probably remove, the possibility of discovering the best possible option.

There is a common misunderstanding that accepting the best option in life can be the result of having no other options. When there is no other option, whatever you are doing feels like a "have to," something imperative, something against your will. You can't make the most serious decision in your life when you feel obligated to only one direction. Choosing the best direction has to include multiple alternatives which aren't chosen.

The fantasy of being kidnapped and forced against your will to become slave illustrates this common misunderstanding. Receiving slave development is an opportunity. If you are forced to undergo the opportunity, then it remains someone else's fault; you can resist like a spoiled brat all the way through the process, and then end up with someone you can blame when it doesn't work out.

That is a common way to go through life. We often try to repeat the patterns we have experienced and exercised throughout our life. That which we fear the most is our strongest prayer. If we fear betrayal, then we subconsciously do everything possible to set up a betrayal so that we can feel we were right about our fears and doubts.

The exercise of anyone else's will against you is the greatest excuse that could ever be found for not taking responsibility for our lives. "It was all the dominant's fault," we want to declare. Leaving us free to say, "I told you so," and to feel good about ourselves while we refuse every option the Universe offers us.

Every day, a slave in development has to feel that he could easily leave the development process. There have to be financial, social and other alternatives that are constantly available during every day of the growth.

A slave cannot continue his development for even one day and still make any progress when he feels that there might be even one other alternative that could be better. When his heart makes him want to explore the alternative, it is imperative that he do so. You can neither go through life nor through slave development constantly might looking over your shoulder at what you think might be better. You have to know that what you are doing is the very best possible route. You have to know that there isn't anything to look over your shoulder for.

Becoming slave requires an internal commitment to achieve unqualified obedience. That doesn't come with any adjustments. It can't at the same time be unqualified and still be negotiable. It can't be unqualified, and yet in place only during convenient times. It can't be unqualified and be felt and experienced only in convenient places.

When you feel you are pursuing the most direct route to your destiny, and are being developed with the highest integrity possible for the highest purpose possible, without egotistic or selfish motivation, then you can develop as a slave. If your plan is to drag your feet through the whole process, then you are planning your failure. If your plan is go through the process because someone is forcing you to, you are planning your failure.

- **YOU CAN'T BECOME FINANCIALLY INVOLVED WITH YOUR OWNER.**

When you have become financially dependent, co-dependent, or even inter-twined, you have lost the independence necessary to feel the required level of honesty. Being connected in a way that there is even an inconvenience to ending the current arrangement places a cost on ending that arrangement.

When the arrangement is with your Owner to develop your slavery, you have killed the chance of becoming slave when you don't have the freedom to honestly express, to pursue other alternatives, or to go back to where you were before you began your development.

Making a financial exchange is a death knell to becoming slave. You don't then know whether it is that exchange that creates the interest in you, or whether it is you personally who is creating the interest. The reality of what is happening doesn't matter. What matters is that you can never know for sure when there is any reason to have a doubt. When you have exchanged anything of substantial value as a condition for beginning your development, you will never be clear, and never be sure, and never be slave.

If you want to get married, then put all your resources into the same pot and live accordingly. If you want to marry a Master, do the same thing. If you want to become slave, then retain your independence and your clarity. There is plenty of time left after you become slave, after you are Born to have a relationship. Don't endanger your slavery by distracting and diverting your energy away from the core issue of becoming who you are. When you know first who you are, then what you do comes from an honest place with integrity, including any resulting relationships.

- **YOU MUST MAINTAIN A SEPARATE LIVING ARRANGEMENT FROM YOUR OWNER.**

Being developed for and accepting your slavery is about your spiritual destiny. Finding the motivation, courage, conviction, strength and internal resources to do only that for which you were created for the rest of your life is the biggest, most challenging process you will ever experience.

Becoming slave also requires experiences which cause you to doubt, and fight against the truth, your nature, the inevitability, and the seriousness of your life. You must have quiet time, private time and peaceful time to make this single most important decision of your life.

When you live with your Owner, you can't help but search for the opportunity to manipulate, criticize, and try to manage the process so that you can avoid the hard questions, the challenging experiences, and the life-giving lessons you need. When you don't have an independent living arrangement, then the Owner's living arrangement is yours, and you egotistically feel as though you must have some say in that arrangement.

If you want to be slave, plan on maintaining a separate household from the Owner. Once slave, then you will live where you are supposed to live. Your egotistic plans to put together the relationship that you can clearly identify as being a good one for you has nothing to do with your becoming slave. Get clear: do you want to become slave, or spend your time trying to implement your expectation of what a Master/slave relationship should be for you? But, don't try to do both, and don't delude yourself into thinking that you can.

- **YOU MUST BE EXPOSED TO THE PUBLIC**

Being honest doesn't mean stopping every person you know on the street and giving them your opinion of them. Telling ugly ladies that they look ugly to you will never strengthen your reputation for being honest.

Being honest, as gays, and as slaves, means being willing to let others know the truth. You don't have to shout the truth, you don't have to take out ads, and you don't have to keep hammering at everyone you know about who you are just because they won't tell you to "shut up" as you keep going on and on about something they're not even interested in.

Being slave is about what you do for the Universe to influence the world. You are never going to be an effective influence if you are closeted, closed off, behind closed doors, or less than proud of who you are. That's not to say that you can't have some influence. Having some influence confirms you have reached the point of being egotistically developed. It is arrogant and incorrect, however, to feel that because you have influence now, that the influence is either adequate or in the right direction to support your destiny. If you could know your destiny before inheriting it, there is no point to inheriting it.

The knowledge of who and how to influence comes from being honest, having integrity, and being only one person to all people. If you feel the necessity to be private and alone in your slavery, and public only about the parts of your life that you are egotistically proud of, you aren't motivated to find your destiny. You can't have it both ways.

You can't have your destiny and then determine if you like it. Destiny is a single path for each person, without any possibility of deviation. Without a complete commitment to following that path, you can never learn of the path. That's the way the world is designed. No one has any control over its design.

Therefore, many of the experiences necessary to achieve your slavery will have to do with being exposed publicly. There you can learn whether or not you really have pride in who you are, because that's the way your Creator made you, or whether you only give lip service to it.

Public experience teaches that your expectation of how people will react is the single most influential determinant of how they *will* react. You will also learn that your expectation of how others react to you is the ceiling for the quality of their reaction. No one can ever react better to you than you do to yourself. If you find yourself apologizing for who you are, they will find doubt and weakness there, and feel invited to attack. Apology, like shame, is an invitation, not an excuse. It encourages criticism, and even provides the behavior that is attacked.

Your public experiences will teach you that you are an example, a model of how to live, whether or not you want to be. We can't switch off and on when we are showing others how we feel people should live and act. Egotistically, most of us would like to believe that we can.

When in public, you have the opportunity to have the influence you should have — there can be real interaction. All the theoretical discussion that you have behind closed doors will never have the slightest effect. The "rubber hits the road" only when you are out in the public doing things. In life, you are either the observer or the observed. We can't be both because of human limitations in our resources.

What you do and when you do it is your Owner's business. He takes orders. Where you end up being,

being seen and being observed are the results of His orders. The purpose of His orders is to give potential slaves the opportunities needed to grow into and qualify for their destinies. You can react either with resistance, or learn the most important lessons of all.

Nothing is more important than learning that we are protected by our Creator only in truth. When we are being, living like, or pretending to be anyone other than who we really are, then we aren't in truth, and we are vulnerable to all the things our egos fear. Only when we accept the truth, without qualification, are we protected, even when we don't know how we could be.

The Universe protects ITs agenda, and preserves ITs investment. When in pursuit of destiny, we are in pursuit of the Universe's investment. In public, we learn that the Universe is present. IT is real, IT is constant, and IT is unrelenting in satisfying all of Its obligations to us as ITs creatures. In private, all the information about life will never be more than intellectual fodder, fun for the mind, and candy for the ego. In public, we learn the truth, how it works, and what we should do with it.

• LIFE MUST BECOME INTEGRATED

The process of becoming slave is a progressive release of everything else except for our slavery. Before we begin slave development, our lives are very compartmentalized. We either intentionally or unintentionally separate our entertainment from work, our gay friends from our business associates, and our family from our personal life. Over and over, every day in every way, we work to maintain that separation because we think that we have to and that it is in our best interest.

The Universe limits what we can egotistically achieve or perform. When IT takes responsibility, and IT always does when we let go of it, there is no need to spend our time and resources in being a different person for different people. The Universe has a plan that will allow us to be whole, to be one person and to have integrity. Only by totally releasing responsibility will the Universe respond. So long as we hold any responsibility, concern or fear about the truth of who we are, the Universe won't manage our lives. IT will let us continue to perform the management of our lives out of the same fears, phobias, weaknesses and limitations that we have always had. The Universe won't fight us for control. Only when we accept our integrity — being only one person — will the Universe do ITs work.

Becoming slave is the process of slowly stepping into the real world of faith. The faith is that the Universe is there, and that IT will act only in our best interest. It would violate our common sense to let go of everything at once. So, we have to let go little by little.

Slaves are given Owners who set up the circumstances, and provide both the power and the impetus to let go. One decision, one step, one compartment at a time, we release our frightfully inadequate and frail ego's locked control over our lives. It is the Owner's job to make us uncomfortable enough to consider letting it go. When you do, the right things happen to confirm our faith and let it grow into a knowing, instead of being only faith.

Integrity demands letting go of the fears that prevent honesty. We don't lie because we think it's the wrong thing to do. We lie because we feel some justification for doing so. That justification is the result of our fears. The explanation for lying is always worded around what we fear would happen if the truth were either told or known. We fear everything and anything that doesn't shed a positive egotistic light on us. Our fear is really of what others will think of us.

• LIFE MUST BECOME LITERAL

One of the ways we get around the truth is by always reading between the lines, even when there is nothing between those lines. Or, by interpreting everything that was said in ways that conform to our prior expectation of what we think should have been said. Another trick is to consider everything an analogy — a story to explain some truth — rather than being the truth itself.

There is no limit to the ways that the ego keeps us from accepting the truth as literal, our orders as being literal, and our lives as being literal. When everything is literal, it is either black or white. The "gray area" is the only place where there is room for the ego to squirm and maneuver so it can continue to do what it is doing now, and what it wants to do.

The purpose of all of life's experiences, and of achieving destiny, is to find moral certainty in every action, and in every moment. The ego rationalizes that so long as there is no black or white, and that only gray exists, then it can never be sure about what to do in any given moment. So long as it maintains that lie, there is no reason for ever trying to reach moral certainty.

If the ego is still arguing for gray, it is still arguing for the impossibility to know order, to know the truth, and to know what must be done, or not done. A slave's general rule for life is "When there is a doubt, do nothing. When there is no doubt, act immediately." Gray says there will never be a time that we are without doubt, and therefore no moral responsibility can ever be taken for our actions.

We want to feel that we are victims in the world. If we feel incapable of ever achieving moral certainty, then we are arguing that we must remain victims. Some victimhood is very obvious and straight-forward. The more complex our thinking, the more complex our interpretation and implementation of victimhood.

So long as we remain victims, we remain without responsibility. So long as "I had no choice" is a believable explanation, we can do whatever we want to do, always and in any circumstance. That is a lie of the highest order. "I had no choice" really means that I wasn't motivated to doing anything different. Motivation is impossible to find if we don't believe in a literal life, where everything is either right or not, and that we can all achieve that knowledge and practice.

It is achievable, however, only after we become honest with ourselves about who we are. So long as we are lying about that, we can never know what is consistent with the truth of who we are.

It is the job of formalized religions, students of ethics, and philosophers to accumulate the general rules of right and wrong. Some come very close to reflecting what is right or wrong. Some are accurate only for the predetermined circumstances that are assumed in their discussion.

The ego would like to "reason" that it is capable of synthesizing, digesting and understanding so completely all the formal rules of the world, and when they apply, that it would never have to submit to the indignity of letting us be who we really are. The ego can't fathom being that far out of control.

When we accept who we are, the rules as they apply to us specifically will be known. Without outside education or influence, exact right and wrong will be known to us. Almost all of what is right and wrong will be the same as the formal moral and ethical rule makers have proposed, because of the integrity of purpose those rule makers have. There will be differences, however, that are just as moral or immoral as those that are published, popular and well known.

Note, too, that they will be accurate only for ourselves. What we learn as being morally correct or incorrect can apply only to us, and never to anyone else. Where the current rule makers have stepped outside their bounds is in believing that what is true for them is true for everyone. It is not. Even though those rules serve a very good purpose by giving us guidelines while we qualify for our destiny, our destiny will replace them, and make them unnecessary.

We have to be literal thinkers. We have to know that we can't rationalize the right to ever do wrong. We have to have the clarity and courage to implement the truth we learn. Common sense will prevent us from accepting or implementing any code of behavior which allows a rationalization that it is okay to have errors, or that we can apply selectively.

Another purpose of the ego is to rationalize that this whole thought about moral certainty is proper, and then add the caveat that it has the right to turn it off and on as it sees fit to accomplish its objectives. Until we know that we have made an immutable decision to never allow the possibility of moral wrong, we won't inherit the wisdom of the truth as it relates to us. We can't collect the information academically, then let the ego decide when it wants to accept it or ignore it.

Becoming slave is a lot about fighting this one issue. Deciding, in obedience, to never have another moral failure for the rest of our lives is too much for the ego to accept. So, we spend a lot of time trying to argue out of it. The literal certainty is the result of complete, unqualified obedience. Qualify the obedience, and you qualify the literal certainty. Qualify the certainty and you qualify the chance of becoming slave.

- INVITE EVERY EXPERIENCE

The ego wants to control what it experiences, so that it can stay in control. The process of slave development is to not control it. When we stop controlling, we are accepting the truth that has always existed. That truth is that we don't really control anything. We delude ourselves into believing that, so life is easier for us, and so we don't have to make the hard decisions about doing what we are supposed to be doing with our lives. So long as we control, we can argue to ourselves that it is all right to continue to pursue what we want to, instead of what was destined for us.

Accepting every experience is the process of the S/M. When we are exposed to the pressure of a device, we have a decision to make about inviting or resisting the experience. When we invite it, we learn that things happen, that we have experiences that we could never imagine. When we resist it, then we experience pain.

When we experience pain, then the ego has the chance to see if it can "process" what is happening. It thinks that either by allowing out-of-body, or by chanting, or by praying, or by some other method that it will be able to "handle" the pressure.

When someone is a slave, he doesn't have to handle what is going on. The pressure takes him where he needs to go, and there, discovers the truth. The only reason to "handle" anything is to avoid the truth, avoid having to experience the truth, and avoid reacting honestly to what happens in the experience.

S/M is a small representation of life. When slave, S/M is a true and honest part of the nutrition by which you live. What is experienced in that short period of time is representative of life in general. The pressure of the S/M is like the chronic reality of life. Just like life is affected by our acceptance or our rejection of it, so is the S/M. When we learn that something lives inside us that is capable of using everything we experience, without any control or influence from us, then we learn the same thing about life.

Life doesn't allow us to choose which experiences we will have. There is no reason to. When we have faith, we know that there is a constant wisdom which guides and creates all those experiences. It is foolish to see that wisdom as anything other than superior to our own meager understanding of things. So, if the superior wisdom presents an experience, what is the advantage of our inferior egotistic conscious wisdom fighting it?

- ## LIFE FOR A SLAVE IS ABOUT OBEDIENCE

A slave was created from the ground up to obey. When he obeys, then he can inherit his purpose, the experiences and all the wisdom needed to lead a great and creative life that is filled with happiness.

Let a slave's life be filled with any motivation other than obedience, and he pays the price for the egotistic indulgence. There is no free lunch, and there is no free egotistic indulgence of any sort in the real world. When you honor your wants and needs, your assessment of what you think should and shouldn't happen, when you decide what should be easy and hard, or how much effort should be put into anything, then you are artificially trying to pump up your ego again.

Obedience is where peace is found. Obedience is where your brilliance and purity is found. Obedience is where your integrity is found. You can't have the results of obedience without being obedient. Most try to understand obedience, and then act as though they don't actually have to obey, because they understand so well how to.

That is foolish, but typical, egotistic reasoning. It is reasoning that continues to try to tell the slave that so long as there is something he doesn't understand, there is an excuse for not achieving the best things in life, and that understanding is the solution to everything. It isn't what you understand. It is only what you do that is important.

It is when we quit understanding, and only pay attention to our obedience, that life begins to change, to become the miracle that we are destined to inherit. Nothing is more important than obedience. Nothing teaches more lessons than growing toward becoming more and more obedient.

Obedience is the Universe's trust in Its creature. Obedience is the distinguishing mark of the destined slave. Obedience is the hallmark and fiber of a slave. Obedience is what and who a slave is. When he knows obedience, then he is qualified to love, to respect, to serve, to teach and to make a difference. Until then, he is still in training.

- ## WHAT SPECIFICALLY CONSTITUTES TRAINING?

When a slave is developing, he is exposed to "sessions" which are formal time to expand, through S/M, the slave's growth. Those sessions have to include time to change the focus from the habitual, noisy outside world, time to experience the S/M, the time to be honest about the experience, then time to sleep on it, and to debrief what has been experienced to gain the maximum value from the experience. That takes a minimum of 16 hours.

Sometimes the experience is one on one, and sometimes it is with brothers. The challenge of developing a slave is in providing experiences which can't be controlled. The diversity, in location, circumstance, attendance, number of men, and any other variable helps provide an experience which isn't as expected nor anticipated. When there is more "surprise" there is more to learn — more adventure and less control.

Slaves need an opportunity to live as, be treated as, and be interacted with as slaves. The public exposure is sometimes that occasion. Sometimes it is by providing the environment in which others can learn. There is no substitute for being in an environment where slavery is not only accepted, but respected. There is also no substitute for what can be learned there. What is learned is never what is expected to be learned. In fact, it has to be what isn't expected, to have any educational content.

Slaves need the opportunity to be a part of larger events. In a new environment, there is energy and focus that can't be controlled, nor anticipated. The newness, the openness and the exposure create another difference that makes a difference.

Slaves need to be found in public places doing non-slave events like a Gay Men's Chorus, or a movie, or dinner, or entertaining someone from out of town. When in an average world with those who live in an average world, the practice of integrity and pride in who you are is available. A slave learns that he has something to teach even those he would least suspect could learn from him.

Slaves need to put what they have already learned to work, helping others decide if they are slave, or to answer their questions. Sometimes we really don't understand our lessons until we try to teach them to someone else. Every opportunity to explain to anyone else who will listen what it is we think we already know is very beneficial, particularly for the one who thinks he knows.

Finally, anything else that the slave would never suspect would furnish him with growth has to be experienced. It might be an experience in church. There might be a family event which forces the growth. There could be something that the slave has done for years, but never before as slave. Repeating the experience with a new awareness provides a lesson that otherwise couldn't be learned.

The ego would like to think that it can control where the learning occurs. And, it tries to control every circumstance in which it ends up being so that there are a minimum of circumstances that aren't controlled. As always, anything the ego wins at causes any person of destiny to lose.

Some experiences are to teach the perfectionists among us the difference between obeying and always being right. Not the same thing. But, it takes an occasion to understand that as perfectionists we do as little as possible that is new or different because in anything new there is the opportunity of making a mistake. Making a mistake is the worst fate that any perfectionist could experience.

Ultimately, being slave is experiencing whatever your Creator wants you to experience. That takes faith, trust and belief in the value of everything the Universe has made. When we move from "lip service" faith, to putting our physical and moral lives on the line for what we believe, we act and react differently. Accepting our destiny is moving the impact of everything we think, say, or do way up the scale. People of destiny can't hide from the impact of their actions. Being Born is to stop spending all your time wanting to.

Finding your destiny is serious business. When that business is about becoming slave, because that's the destiny you have been created with, there are a lot of people involved in helping you achieve that destiny.

What happens during slave development is exactly what needs to happen to satisfy that serious business. Every belief has to be sacrificed so that you can experience the truth without the constraint that current belief causes. After achieving the willingness to let go of every belief, then you must have every experience necessary to confirm the new set of beliefs.

Since the new beliefs are acquired through experience, they are held with deeper and more passionate force. That passion will make the slave effective in the execution of his destiny. Anything less and he is simply imitating life instead of living it.

Expect anything that you can't expect nor anticipate. Expect it to be different from what you have heard others have gone through. Expect it to be unique to you, and to be designed to provide only your destiny. Anything less, and you end up with nothing more than the ego you started out with.

The process of accepting destiny is very similar to that of becoming airborne as a pilot. On the ground there are certain laws of physics at work. As soon as the aircraft has left the ground virtually everything changes.

When an aircraft is on the ground it can be steered by turning the wheels. There is no vertical freedom; everything must be accomplished in a two-dimensional plane. Most important, just like being in a car, when everything else fails you can simply step on the brakes and everything will come to a halt in a matter of seconds.

Once airborne, however, not only is maneuvering accomplished in a two dimensional plane, but also up and down. Other aircraft have to be avoided in three dimensions, and turning is a matter of setting up an arc against the air that produces the turn. Most different, however, is that there are no brakes. In a plane, if something happens, if things get out of control, it could be a portion of an hour, compared to seconds on the ground, before things can be brought to a halt. A landing site must be selected. If there is no power, there is no second chance to land. The site and the approach must be carefully calculated because there is no room for mistakes. Everything is in terms of doing the right thing next, instead of simply applying the brakes to make everything stop.

When we accept our destiny, life becomes about determining what comes next. The option to stop, to hold back, to resist is gone. Knowing the spiritual world, trusting IT, and the wisdom and instincts which come from IT is the information on which we must depend for the next action. We have to trust, and don't have time to analyze, to figure out, to understand, or to produce an acceptable alternative. What is happening is all that is happening.

The challenge is seeing without bias the truth in every situation. Then, it is knowing there is no black spot on our soul that could motivate us to take action for the wrong reason or purpose.

If any of the conditions are missing, then we crash, just like when in the air. The ego tells us that we can always apply the brakes. In real life there are no brakes. It is only after the brakes have been applied that we have time to "think about things." Without brakes there is no such time. Thinking about things is a luxury which the ego enjoys, but has nothing to do with living. It is egotistic entertainment. Understanding serves its purpose only in helping others. Our own life isn't the result of understanding. It is the result of not understanding. It is the result of obeying.

A slave's life is the result of having experienced the truth, accepting it and living accordingly, and practicing the truth experienced in obedience. So it is with every person of destiny. Getting there is what happens during slave development.

Additional Thoughts on Development of slave

SlaveMaster:

I've begun slave development with men who have searched for as much as 25 years for their slavery, only to discover within 20 minutes that they aren't slave at all and have been pursuing something that isn't authentic for them for most of their lifetimes. Others have ended the process because they recognized that the slave development was about to let them know, through direct experience, for certain whether or not they are slave. Others are more subtle and make excuses for why not to continue their development so they can avoid the Truth and consequences of their destiny.

If I am using S/M to develop a slave and order it to provide no feedback, I am taking responsibility for doing so, and claiming that I know better than it, what is safe and what it needs. That is as it should be. However, if I'm not ready to take that responsibility I must order feedback when that is what I need to be responsible.

The human ego cannot even imagine the order, the satisfaction or the potential that it releases when the destined Owner/slave connection is made. Life begins at a point beyond what the ego could dream possible, and it grows from there.

A slave's greatest, and only real, responsibility is where it places its obedience. So long as a slave is still asking the question, "Should I Obey?" (Capitalization intentional) it should not be obeying. Instead, it should be learning, growing and exploring. Instead, it should be either preparing for its current Master who might one day spiritually qualify to become its Owner, or preparing for the day it will find its rightful, destined Owner. During this development period a slave should be only agreeing, considering its options, reviewing the benefits of its current relationship, and constantly examining if it should continue.

slave 7:

Obedience is always primary, but so is the lack of self-control in a slave. You cannot control your own slave development, and a slave doesn't become urge-less by some sort of massive self-control. Rather, it is the allowing of the real slave inside to merely be what it is, which requires that the consciousness not control it. And the slave can't do this in isolation. The Master must be there to control that slave being when it comes to the fore. Otherwise, it is unsafe.

You were either born (at the time of biological birth) with a slave spirit or you were not. The process of slave development only reveals that truth. Slavery is not something one accomplishes; it is not something one strives for. Simply strive to be your truest self via obedience to your authentic spirit, and life takes care of itself. Slavery is easy when the slave realizes that all it is doing is being its "self," true to nature, true to spirit. And being ourselves is easy, once we have cleaned off all the gunk that accumulates over the years, which is often an arduous process, and begin to feel "connected" to Something we hadn't felt before. Being Born is not an end, but rather a new beginning. The journey of growth through life is never-ending, or should be.

Ego

SlaveMaster:

The ego can remain in control, be unthreatened, and remain our premiere self-identification.

Only the ego is arrogant enough to try to accomplish being connected, to gain the benefits, and then turn around and try to take claim to and credit for those benefits. The only claim I can make is to the quality and consistency of My obedience. Everything else IS a gift — purely, clearly and completely.

An absolute freedom from what others think comes from being connected. Having others disagree with My experiences is, at most, an amusement that comes from remembering being devoid of My connection and so sure of My erroneous egotistic views back then. The same freedom from taking credit for what I do is a freedom from criticism. None of My actions or words is Me, and none of it is Mine. Try to claim it, and the Universe will stop giving the commands that allow IT to accomplish Its tasks through Me. The Universe cannot be misled into believing I obey when I don't, just so I can get orders which I could then abuse. We cannot abuse the privilege of being given orders, the privilege of being connected. If we do, the orders will stop.

slave 7:

Being subjected to abuse as a child seems to be the main thing that helped this slave know the distinction between the false self and real self at an early age. Somehow, this slave had the wherewithal to sit back and really observe as a kid. Trauma often seems to kick people into the realm of the very real and out of the more superficial concerns of the ego. Throughout adulthood, this slave has been able to access/consult/know the heart (the real self) when the chips were really down and something important was transpiring. This is not to say that to this day 7 doesn't have its ego issues. it does. Still, its ego may create emotions within, but it rarely causes a real action.

It can be confusing as to what a desire of the ego is and what is a desire or need of the real self. For whatever reason, in 7 the real self simply seems to be more powerful than the ego... and experience tells 7 that the real self brings joy while the ego brings emotional pain. If one simply lives and observes that the ego is what is causing emotional pain, then that is what guides one in staying away from the ego.

7 is not exempt from having an ego. It creeps up and creates concerns that it knows are not real. We cannot control our emotions nor always the rise of the ego, but we can choose in advance to recognize them and deal with them appropriately.

How does one release the ego to surrender and obey? Oh, the billion-dollar question. If anyone could answer that for you, you would not have a life. At least, that is how this slave looks at it. The journey of life is making it to the point where one can feel that the ego is not driving. Generally, though, this slave believes there is no "HOW?" One just stumbles along, or floats downstream, until one is there. Over the course of this slave's life, it noticed those experiences that gave it a clue that there is something within worth trusting, and it is not the ramblings nor the logical thinking of the mind. The more one notices such a thing inside, the more one can let go and trust it.

This slave has never once been angry with its Master. Anger would seem to be an ego issue, or something telling about how the Master and slave do not connect.

WHAT IS THE EMOTIONAL PATH?
An Article by SlaveMaster

Originally, it takes courage to consider slavery, because it sounds to us like it is so far from the ordinary. And, first off, anyone who doesn't feel successful isn't even qualified to become a slave, because being slave is the final and highest level of consciousness; it is the acceptance of destiny.

It is easy to give everything up when there isn't anything to give up. It is, however, a real challenge to risk anything when everything is going well for you, everything except for being who you are, and everything except for having your integrity.

Once the courage is found to begin the pursuit of slavery, a method to begin has to be discovered. Some advertise and spend a night or a weekend at a time with someone who has mutual interests in providing the slave environment. Others pay for the experience by the hour from professionals. Others research, and find a safe and supportive environment for a weekend where they can be with many others at the same time, such as at Butchmann's Academy.

When those who are slave are first exposed to authentic slavery, when they have a chance to experience and consider slavery as a possible life, there is a tremendous elation and a tremendous release. The hole in our life that has become bigger and bigger over time feels as though it might have a "cure." It feels as though there might really be a solution to what is missing from our life.

- Phase 1: Acknowledging that there is something real and satisfying in our lives that has been suppressed by our self-control.

Our lives are a tremendous investment. A lot of bumps and bruises, many attempts and failures and, finally, personal, ego-driven success has been experienced. We deny ourselves the easy way to make it to success. We do what those we respect have told us to do to achieve. We do many things that no one else has supported us in, but that worked out anyway. The success is our pride.

If we are healthy, it doesn't feel as if the effort was wasted. There might be some regrets. We might have gone without a childhood. We might have denied our gay sexuality. We might have lived like we were straight, without even the enjoyment of our fetishes or non-standard heterosexual passions. We have acted ordinary, when we aren't.

When the light starts coming in the window, it feels wonderful. We think we are through having to experience anything negative. We hope that it will all be downhill from here. We feel we might have reached the end of trials and tribulations. Life is now going to be as easy as putting on a pair of handcuffs; easier, because someone else will put them on.

- Phase 2: Realizing we have to let go of our facades and the images we have built.

It has taken a long time to realize our current success. It has hurt us to have to live in the slave closet and keep up the smiles and faked excitement in our lives while our secret interests have haunted us. It seems like good news that we can let go of all of that.

When we start to let go of that which we thought we hated doing for all these years, something strange happens. We learn that the lies and deceit protected us.

Our pride is even, partially, a product of how well we were able to manage the unmanageable. It's uncomfortable for us to let go of what we thought we detested or disliked doing. It has become a part of who we think we are.

The people who know and love us have come to expect a certain consistency from us. If we begin to change, we rationalize that it will undermine the security that others feel from us because we are so predictable. Even if we can face our own fears regarding the loss of a self- image that we have come to respect along with others who have come to respect us, we reason that we must hold on to the lies for the family and friends we have accumulated and developed over time.

We find an internal objection to doing what we thought we have wanted to do all our life. It isn't as simple as we expected. It requires overcoming even more challenges that all those that made us successful, and in which we take such pleasure and satisfaction.

- Phase 3: We are faced with making the biggest decision of our life.

The most basic of all sales theories is that we buy when the reasons to buy outweigh the reasons not to. Like any balance scale, we collect the reasons to buy on one side of the scale and the reasons not to on the other. When making a decision, we collect the reasons to proceed on one side of the scale and the reasons not to on the other.

The reasons to become slave include because it opens us up to a part of our lives that has been hidden and suppressed. Other reasons are that it provides an improved environment from which we can sexually express ourselves, and that it gives us a way to belong, to feel a part of a community that is more specifically ours.

On the "reasons not to buy" side, we know that it is going to change our life. All change has associated stress. Everyone we know is going to have to change their perception of us, decide whether they are now going to accept us, and many are going to criticize us. Life is never going to be the same, and we don't know how it is going to be. There will be more unknown than known.

The further we get into the process of identifying both the reasons to become slave and the reasons not to become slave, we find that there are many reasons not to. Finally, we see the list of reasons to become slave is relatively short, and that many of those reasons sound selfish.

- Phase 4: Recognizing that there isn't sufficient reason to become slave without a strong belief in the spiritual imperative of life.

There isn't enough fun, excitement or sexual satisfaction to justify giving up our current life for slavery. There has to be a bigger reason to become slave. What we naively associate with being slave can be acquired on the weekend, from those who are also satisfied by giving their attention and interest for two days without feeling any responsibility for the remainder of the slave's life.

Every conceivable benefit won't raise the stakes to the point that giving your life to slavery is worthwhile without adding to that list the fulfillment of our created purpose. There are many other alternatives such as becoming a regular S/M practitioner, or finding a lover who likes to play. If we aren't ready to give our life to slavery, we can't become slave. It isn't that we become poor slaves, we don't become slaves at all.

- Phase 5: Accepting that being slave is about unqualified obedience.

Slavery can occur only after all limitations of what will be done with our lives, and which areas of our life will be released to the authority we recognize, are eliminated. There is no such thing as partial slavery. We live as we must live, in moral certainty, and without the possibility of moral failure, or our slavery isn't granted to us. Our slavery remains a moving target that we can't reach without unqualified surrender to obedience.

The Universe is the only decider of who and when someone becomes slave. No man has ever been entrusted with that decision. Neither the man who might be slave, nor the one who develops him can decide that someone will now be slave. No one will ever become slave by accident, prematurely, or in error. Obedience is doing what the Universe wants us to do. We have to recognize that life isn't about us, and never was. And, of course, it never will be.

The confusion occurs when we try to take credit for the spiritual investment the Universe has made in us. The spirit can't act through us until we are qualified to have it work through us. So, it has given us the education, I.Q. and environmental influences necessary to become qualified.

If, after becoming qualified by the spirit, we egotistically claim credit for all that the spirit has done for us, we have pride we don't deserve, and we act as though we are trying to steal the result of the spiritual investment. We have no such right, and it should be no surprise that life is difficult and unfulfilling when we are egotistic and in pursuit of what we egotistically want.

Accepting our destiny, becoming obedient, surrendering or not, are the only real choices we have. It is a question of letting the spirit have its purpose.

Are you going to give the spirit its purpose? Is it worth it?

It is the only question that matters, and it will be the hardest decision to make. When you feel you have more to gain than to lose, you will proceed with your slavery. So long as you feel you have more to lose than you have to gain, you won't proceed. It's that simple, and that straight-forward.

The answer comes in knowing the value and purpose of the spirit. The pursuit of slavery is the experience of all the right things we need to experience to gain sufficient information to make this one, single decision.

Look forward to, and invite into your life, everything, so that you will finally know what you need to know to decide what to do with your spirit's life.

Fantasy

slave 7:

This slave's experiences tell it that fantasy may propel us on, but once fantasy becomes expectation or demand, it then limits us, and we stand a good chance of missing an unexpected and more wonderful reality.

Fear

SlaveMaster:

Most of us go on and on through life complaining about being frustrated at not having the life we want. The reason we do is because it is easier to complain than it is to face the fear of being who we were designed to be, without any control or influence over who that is.

I've personally taken seven men to a benchmark in their spiritual evolution which I refer to as Birth, and have taken more than 300 from one step in their evolution to the next. What becomes clear from that experience is that fear of knowing for sure whether or not they are slave, and accepting the consequences of that awesome Truth is the single biggest stopping point to accepting slavery.

slave 7:

While many slaves feel fear and even anger, 7 has (since meeting SlaveMaster and beginning slavery) never had a moment's fear or hesitation, has never looked for a way out. Every further step 7 takes into slavery, it feels tremendous joy and celebrates, as life energy seems to burst forth from within. 7 is a very lucky thing.

There is nothing to fear in a Born slavery that is right and true. The slave will experience the want that the Owner wants, and the two will be as One, act as One, and match in desire as One.

Fear is there for a reason, and one needs to pay attention to it. Fear often needs to win. There is no strength in overcoming a legitimate fear.

Force

SlaveMaster:

Mastery-slavery is a pure and natural state of existence, and both Masters and slaves must grow to accept and embrace this calling. Without full acceptance and embrace, then there is no reason at all to pursue Mastery-slavery.

slave 7:
A slave who requires force:
- Would prefer to be a victim rather than a slave.
- Does not wish to give the gift of slavery to its Master.
- Retains the right to say no
- Doesn't have to take any responsibility for who and what it is.
- Maintains separation between Master and slave.
- Can be a slave and pretend not to be, in the heart and soul.
- Never has to accept who it is deep down.

Some think that without force there is no real slavery, but they are using a definition of slavery we are not.

Force (in ways you imagine being forced) is fantasy and play. Force means rejecting Master's affections, powers, and goodness. Force means the slave may wish to take the shortcut to slavery, rather than go through the process of self discovery and growth. If one is slave (or Master), then one feels it as a calling that will not cease. The yearning is deep and all-encompassing.

Force from a Master perspective:

- Your slave rejects You, and refuses to accept You.

- Master gets no gifts from the slave, but only steals.

- Your slave has told You that you are not worthy.

- Master gets no honor or pride of Ownership.

- Your gifts of Mastery have been rejected by the slave.

- Your slave is not giving You gratitude and affection.

- Force means a hell of a lot of work for no real benefit.

SlaveMaster only begins with someone He truly believes is slave at heart. He only begins when He feels there is enough readiness in the slave. He only continues if He and the slave both recognize a real connection between them. He provides experiences that are in the best growth interests of His slave, rather than follow His own wishes. He is always obedient to His true self and to the connectedness He feels to the Universe, which creates consistency and trust for the slave. The trust he creates leads to the safety the slave spirit needs so that it can come out and live. And then He waits (and waits and waits and waits) until the slave heart presents itself fully to and for Him.

It is this slave's experience that if one is to live as slave by consent, then one gives in slavery; one does not need or take coercion. Likewise, the Master is also giving, not taking. And in this mutual giving, both receive the sense of an honest life fully-lived.

Freedom in Slavery

slave 7:

Whereas some may classify living with SlaveMaster as intense, for 7 being His slave is calming, soothing, and peaceful. "Intense" is how 7 classifies all the years it lived before meeting SlaveMaster: intense yearnings, intense emptiness, intense dissatisfaction with life, and intense stress created by the inability to live as its gut told it to live. For 7, freedom is now in slavery. The lack of freedom is what it experienced all the years before meeting SlaveMaster. Now, it has the freedom to be totally itself, pure and unhampered by many of the trappings of life that we all fall into. Restlessness is what characterized most of 7's life prior to its actualization of slavery. Peace and freedom is what it has now. it is Home.

Mastery is not domination. Rather, it is the creation of the safety and the set of experiences the slave needs to feel the time and place is right to let go of the slave desires already within. Master doesn't make a slave. He only creates the environment in which the slave will happily reveal itself to Him.

"I own your thoughts," He may say with the intention of letting you (His slave) know that you may tell Him anything at all, that you needn't worry about secrets or about how to approach Him. "I own your thoughts," can be an expression of His openness to hear and know and honor everything about you. "The only thing you will ever do in life is obey!" indicates that you will have total freedom from concern and the burdens of worry and choice. "A slave has no rights to anything but obedience!" only furthers His stance that you will be free in that He will take such complete and caring responsibility for you that you have no reason to be concerned about your rights. All you have to do is be true to your Heart.

It also occurs to this slave that slaves have the "good life" while Master's have the responsibilities, and yet who are the ones who seem to resist it all the most?

It seems to this slave that the slave gets SO MUCH more joy and pleasure than the Master. Being slave can be a long-lasting erotic joyride.

This slave just imagined a conversation between itself and a layperson who was outraged and aghast at the concept of slavery. She said, "How horrible! Being required to do things against one's will!" To which this slave replied: "Correction: being required to do things *for* one's will."

Born slavery is a natural unity of two or more who have let go of the choices and power they only thought they had, and have embraced the flow of energy that runs through them, letting that energy decide, guide, motivate, love, create, empower...

Growth

SlaveMaster:

Slavery is all about growth. The desire, the need and the enjoyment of obeying is the motivation to grow. Owned or not, the growth must be continuous. Don't egotistically be distracted by finding "Mr. Right" Owner when there are personal growth opportunities still available. As the law of nature states, "Anything not growing is dying."

We each are where we are right now and we each need to grow.

Everything between natal birth and a slave finding its rightful qualified owner is about growth. Because we're growing, something should look different every day from the way it looked the day before.

While we are frustrated at what is not happening, there are lessons in front of us that are preventing us from moving to the next step in our life because we are too distracted to learn the current lesson. When we're having trouble finding new work, it is because we have yet a lesson to learn in the current job. When we can't find a new relationship, it is because we have some unfinished business in another relationship.

Fortunately or unfortunately, almost all of life's lessons are learned from experiencing what doesn't work. The only way to develop confidence, and to proceed through life with passion, is to
know for certain that all the other alternatives result in failure. What is left over is what does work, and what we dedicate our lives to. No one else can tell us what won't work. We have to find out on our own, through personal experience. There is no substitute for experience. The parental urge to give others the answers to life before they learn it through the school of hard knocks is hard to overcome. None of us will ever do anything really significant in life that hasn't been empowered through experience. That makes the job of being an Owner or Master one of providing those growth experiences, not of providing answers.

Our collective and individual task is to facilitate life's processes for each other so that we go through life's phases as quickly as possible while those who understand and support us in an unqualified, non-judgmental way are witnessing what we do.

We grow through life. Things only make sense when we have certain beliefs already in place from education or experience. Once a lesson is learned, we are free to change beliefs to prepare for the next lesson.

When I was "growing up," I didn't have mentors, peers, advisors or others to model My life after. I didn't have anyone who could help and to whom I could tell My truth. I'm privileged to be a part of changing that which would have made a difference while I was discovering and growing.

By telling the truth as fast as we can, without shame, embarrassment or hesitation we can facilitate each other's growth, while helping ourselves learn where we are and determine what we should do next.

Our task in life is to learn where we are, express openly and freely what we're having difficulties with, and to review what others have done to achieve their growth by getting past each challenge. All of us have something more to learn, and some of us may be very adult in one area of our lives but still struggling with getting through other areas.

Regardless of where we are, that's where we need to WANT to be.

Contemplating where we are now is critical to knowing who we really are, what we should be learning now, and what might be coming next.

slave 7:

Growth is really a trip back to once was, before it all got derailed. Growth is a trip back to one's self, an oft-forgotten self, a self not well known, a self one is happy being.

"I and It"

SlaveMaster:

When My first slave (slave 1) was near being Born, it came back from its acceptance repeatedly each time it got close to declaring and defining itself as slave through its commitment to obedience. Finally, the slave who become My first-Born said to Me, "Each time I find myself in the state of mind where I'm ready to jump into the reality of who I am, I feel as though I am lying in declaring ownership of myself." Each time the slave declared, "I am slave," it felt the dishonesty of egotistically claiming what never has belonged to itself.

We agreed it would never again refer to itself as "I" or "me," and instead would know itself only as "This slave" (properly capitalized at the beginning of a sentence). When the next opportunity was empowered, that slave was Born. Immediately the slave said that it finally was consciously in the same environment as it was spiritually when it internally declared and permanently and profoundly accepted its slavery.

When the conscious mind was inconsistent with what was experienced, the inconsistency absolutely prohibited advancement. When the slave talked one way, self-identified egotistically, it could not accept the inconsistent and different world of slavery where there is no egotistic self ownership.

Each of the succeeding six slaves were trained to speak the truth, referring only to "This slave" and secondarily as "it." Each graduated to the spiritual benchmark of Birth which confirmed the accuracy of the conscious use references which claimed no egotistic possession.

The spirit and mind must operate consistently for integrity and integration to occur. Forcing the self-reference of "I" and "me" sets up a block to belonging and obeying. It isn't coincidental that several American military organizations force the use of "This marine" or "This soldier" and deny the use of self-reference. Similarly, many religious practices deny the same egotistic reference. As we speak, we think. As we think, we live. As we live, we become. There is clear cause and effect.

The slaves who have responded to the question of protocol unanimously "like" the non-personal protocol because they know it is true, and that any other reference is equally false. A false reference forces a slave to be dishonest, a characteristic they universally abhor and detest. Using a lower case "i" doesn't make it any more honest. Lower case simply makes it apologetic.

slave 7:

For the Owner, the body of the slave is His machine to operate and live in. This is why SlaveMaster calls His slaves "it" rather than any human pronoun. A slave is an "it" — a flesh-and-blood machine that is animated by His life energy, His soul.

7 meets slaves that have trouble with the term "slave." 7 meets Masters who resist being called "Master." But no matter what the ego says, the spirit seeks those who see It for what it really is. 7 is an "it," and SlaveMaster sees that.

Integrity

slave 7:

What kinds of skills should a slave develop in order to be an attractive prospective slave? No skills, but rather the qualities of unfailing integrity and seeking of the Truth.

Intuition

slave 7:

The only thing this slave ever did right was remain true to self: to have a sense of that soft voice within, or intuition, and always follow it. And that really sums up all SlaveMaster is saying: find yourself, know yourself, and obey that self.

Joy

slave 7:

A slave to the right Master, a body without an independent self. The result is not an automaton, but rather a free and spontaneous creature living in accord with its nature. It may seem paradoxical, but obedience has enabled this slave to become joyful and to feel free and pure.

Some may conclude that this slave lives in some sort of blissful state all day long. This is definitely not true. it still feels the 'burdens' of everyday life and has times of frustration and impatience. The eroticism and joy of its slavery to and Oneness with SlaveMaster are always within reach, however.

KINDS OF SLAVES
An Article by SlaveMaster

For more than twenty years I have been dealing with all kinds of slave. Each called itself "slave," and each Master and everyone else referred to each slave as "slave," even when there were vast differences between them.

The confusion arises because whenever anyone speaks about slaves or slavery, each is telling the truth about the kind of slavery being experienced, while each is talking about a different type of slave. Each is telling the truth of their own experience, but it is a different experience nevertheless.

To the listener, what is heard appears to be conflicting information when, in fact, what is being told is a story or a conclusion about something different from what another is speaking about.

I have observed through many slaves with whom I have worked, three distinctly different types of slaves. It is extremely important to recognize that one type is not inherently better or worse than any other type. The best type is the type that is true, that is honest, and that is in integrity with the one who is exploring it. All of us were created different. That, of course, is the fiber and texture of the world which prevents it from being boring — not that anyone who is dealing with consensual, adult slavery has been bored with either the subject or the pursuit!

One of My created purposes is to help those considering slavery identify who they are, and determine whether the pursuit is genuine for them. It has been helpful to be able to quickly refer to a type of slave to facilitate clear thinking and efficient communication on the subject. The objective has led to naming the types of slave I have encountered. The title I have assigned to each is, of course, arbitrary. The point is simply to provide a consistent, quick reference.

- TYPE THREE SLAVE:

Such a slave uses slavery as an alternative form of entertainment. In everyone's life there need to be an activity which relieves the stress, the obligation, and the responsibility of everyday living. The more family, professional or other commitments we have accepted, the more need there is for a time and place of release. Some use massage. Others go to a movie. Some meditate. And, there are those who arrange for a night of a weekend of being slave. The S/M activity of slavery diverts the attention, focuses the thought, and frees the spirit temporarily, and peace and tranquility can then be experienced. The experience prepares us for another day in the world that demands so much.

- TYPE TWO SLAVE:

For this kind of slave, slavery has a priority. There are many things that are important to its life, and slavery is among those things that matter a lot. The slave seeks a profession, recognizes and maintains its family responsibilities, and seeks and negotiates Master/slave relationships which are educational and fulfilling. Like the work the slave performs, each relationship might last for only a few weeks, or it might last the greater part of a lifetime. Also, like the work, the first relationship is seldom the last. There is growth and personal clarity that come from being Mastered by each different person. The slave chooses its Master, and is usually the one who makes the decision to end the Master/slave relationship. This is probably the most common type of slavery to which most are referring when slavery is spoken of, and the type with which most Masters associate.

- TYPE ONE SLAVE:

This is a slave of destiny, because the Owner cannot be negotiated. Connecting to the Owner is like an orphaned child who is seeking its genetic father or mother. Who that parent is cannot be shopped for or negotiated. Who the Owner is was determined before the slave was conceived, as part of the spiritual plan the slave spirit negotiated. This type of slave may or may not live with its Owner, and when it has a Master, it is by assignment from the slave's Owner.

It is conceivable that she same person could be both Owner and Master, and, admittedly, most Masters interchangeably refer to themselves as Owner and Master without distinction. Since I only deal with TYPE ONE slaves, it has been important to me to make a clear differentiation between Master and Owner, to enable easy and clear communication.

Only the actual process of slave development can fully disclose and confirm the type of slave any one individual is designed to be. However, a method I have recommended to many is to close the eyes and imagine a life of only obeying, in every matter and in every way, without option. If that brings a feeling of peace and tranquility to the body, and maybe even brings physical pleasure, there is a clue found about the need to be owned. Similarly, if it brings stress and discomfort to the body, also notice that.

Whatever type of slave anyone is, the path to fulfillment is going to be through being honest and authentic to whatever type each is. The process, then, is one of discovery of the truth. When being slave is treated like a decision, instead of an adventure to uncover what is real, there is the danger of not doing that which is right for the individual. Believing the type of slave someone is results from choice would imply that everything can work just as well either way, slave or not, no matter what is decided. That is not the way it works, and is not the way anyone I know has ever experienced it.

For most involved in modern consensual slavery, the pursuit of slavery is one of life's processes. As such, there are no cookie-cutter approaches nor pat answers to anything. Even what appears to be true at any point in our lives can change. Remember when we truly believed in Santa Claus and the tooth fairy? We acted in integrity, based on those beliefs, then moved on to claim new beliefs.

The process of being slave, and becoming what you are, will follow the same patterns of life that our other growth and development go through. Edison was destined to invent the light bulb. As a teenager, however, he didn't live his life accordingly. The reality and the implications of what he was to do later couldn't be implemented until that later time had arrived.

Be patient, be adventuresome, and know that today's beliefs won't be tomorrow's beliefs. Life is not an academic pursuit, and even knowing the future wouldn't allow us to skip the present. Pursue slavery accordingly. Examine today's truth and live according to that. Be open to tomorrow's truth, and let life change to adjust to the change in belief.

To all types of slaves, know that being slave is authentic and legitimate. If your interest didn't serve some real purpose in your life, you wouldn't be questioning, reviewing or examining the implications. The more accurate the thinking during this adventure, the more rewarding the results will be.

THE NATURE OF KNOWING
An Article by SlaveMaster

We don't know anything for sure. Every scientific understanding is a theory. Yet, we design bridges, travel through space and use the internet without any proof of knowing. I can't prove the sun will come up again tomorrow to start another day, that the next switch I flip will turn on a light, or that My vehicle will start the next time I turn the key. Yet, I live comfortably in this world without being able to confirm knowing any of these things.

Cognitive dissonance is defined as "experience which doesn't match expectation." Only the ego has expectation. Get rid of the ego, and none of the nasty results of failed expectation can occur. Hold onto expectation, and the nasty results must continue. Having expectations produces cognitive dissonance, guaranteed. We have to be insane to expect otherwise.

The point of life is to find out what's authentic inside. We must not confuse authenticity with ultimate "Truth." These are not related concepts. We only have a human mind with which to know. To think we have the ultimate truth requires the arrogance that there is no greater mind in the universe than ours. Being authentic is not related to knowing anything but ourselves. Being authentic, the only source of happiness, is about being honest with ourselves regarding our reactions to the experiences of life. Anyone who has ever believed in Santa Claus has already believed lies to learn life's lessons effectively. Combining knowledge of Truth with being authentic is as artificial as putting "religious right" and "authenticity" together. We believe what we MUST believe to learn what we must learn. Believe nothing and we learn nothing. Believing nothing is very comforting for perfectionists since we then never make the mistake of believing something that is later found to be untrue. Believe something, and we have the opportunity to learn what we need to learn, which forces us to let go of each belief as experience teaches us something new.

Since expectation is a function of the ego, the decision we all have to make about our lives is, "Is the purpose of life to have accurate expectations, or to be authentic and, therefore, happy?" This is a mutually exclusive choice. Good luck to anyone who expects to be the first person in history to answer "both."

The biggest human trap is to pretend we can understand through psychology. The spirit and Truth do not conform to such human theories, nor can they be explained with those theories. To experience, then try to classify and explain, and then to further institutionalize what was learned, is not spiritual. Psychology is very effective at curing the mentally sick, at getting past egotistic patterns that lock us, unnaturally, into a prison that isn't healthy for us. There is a big difference between getting un-sick and growing spiritually.

The question about cognitive dissonance is a question about how getting un-sick will make one grow into authenticity. There is no more correlation than "How does overcoming the mumps further my authenticity?" One doesn't relate to the other, and trying to make them relate is a dead end that is useless and futile to pursue.

Our health and growth will be measured by how rapidly we change our beliefs so we can grow, and how easily we relinquish the old beliefs that no longer serve us, to make room for the next belief. There is no Santa Claus, AND I bless my parents for My thinking there was. I am both proud that I believed in Santa, and unashamed and unapologetic that I no longer do. I now have room for another productive belief, true or not.

With no greater reason than experience, I KNOW the sun will come up tomorrow; I don't just believe it will. I don't care if I'm right or wrong. My life is going to be far more productive because I act as though it is a sure thing, despite all the legitimate arguments that it is not. However, if the sun fails to come up even one day, I will quickly change My KNOWING and dramatically adjust My life to accommodate the new experience.

That is the nature of belief and knowing.

slave 7:

Experience. We can only know from what we experience. And experiences come whenever they come. We can only invite them. We can't make them happen.

Knowledge

slave 7:

Should a slave make itself knowledgeable about the type of fetishes it becomes involved in, for the sake of safety concerns, and how should a slave's concerns and knowledge be pointed out to a Master? This slave's main fetish has always been slavery itself, the concept of being OWNED. So, this slave made itself knowledgeable about slavery itself... the psychology of, the emotional healthiness of, the real life repercussions of... This slave also looked into the physical safety of the things it saw itself doing as slave.

Limits

slave 7:

SlaveMaster says a slave must have no limits. A slave having no limits eliminates the possibility of negotiation between slave and Master and shows the slave's readiness for whatever Destiny brings. Acceptance: no want, no sense of control, no limits.

Losing Self

slave 7:

A slave does not lose itself through obedience. Rather, it embraces itself. Obedience in a growing slave can be seen as a kind of cleansing process, washing away that which has tarnished the spirit during life and revealing the most authentic self within. A Born slave doesn't lose itself or become a blank slate for Master to fill; it finds itself. As SlaveMaster says: what is authentic stays; what is not authentic leaves.

Maintaining Born slavery

slave 7:

It maintains Born slavery through strict Obedience to slave Protocol, strict Obedience to the Will of SlaveMaster that it feels, "hears" or senses when not in SlaveMaster's presence, and prayer (giving thanks to the Universe and 7's Owner) and meditation.

It does not really relapse. 7 does have its ups and downs, its times when it feels completely connected to its Owner and times when it can't feel the connection at all, but 7 has never gone off course nor really relapsed. it does feel rather down if it can't feel the connection to its Owner and can't sense His Will or Presence within, but 7 craves that connection and seeks to re-establish it, via prayer and Protocol. It doesn't always work, however, so there are occasional short periods in which 7 feels like it is just plodding through its waking hours.

7 feels such bliss in its slavery and prior to slavery never thought life much worth living, so "relapsing" is very

unattractive, and rejection of anything the ego may come up with rather easy. Also, allowing its ego any room to try and claim any authority or true self just feels wrong, dishonest and unfaithful to the Universe as well as SlaveMaster.

MASTER vs. OWNER
An Article by SlaveMaster

I feel a need here to distinguish between "Master" and "Owner." The title has no value beyond communicating accurately through shared semantics. The distinguishing characteristic of an Owner is that of making a lifetime commitment to a slave, limited only by the slave's continued willingness to obey.

Many Masters who use the title "Master" have actually made a lifelong commitment, but don't use the word "Owner," mostly because there is no need to do so. Some use the term Master but have little idea what the word means. I've heard the expression in our community of "a 13-minute Master," meaning someone who begins his Master career with the filling-out of an online bio and completes it by pressing the SUBMIT key. The title applies to many with very different purposes and qualifications.

Some use "Master" and "Owner" interchangeably, which isn't sufficient in a discussion of Born slavery. A Master is formally defined as "a person with the ability or power to use, control or dispose of something. A further definition is "a person eminently skilled in something." Those definitions would imply that the use of "Master" in the community is accurate.

The distinction is, singularly, the lifelong commitment an Owner makes without regard to location, relationship, profession, or personal use of his slave. An Owner can also be a slave's Master, when the slave's destined life is closely-enough aligned with the personal purpose of the Owner, often characterized by the slave living full-time in the Owner's environment.

Therefore, a Master can be an Owner, without using the title, and an Owner can also be a Master. The difference between what is meant by "Master" and "Owner" is determined by a review of the level of commitment, and the nature of the never-ending responsibility for a slave. It is imperative that "Owner" be clearly understood in reviewing what is written here about Born slaves and the development process and environment in which such creatures must be nurtured to become empowered with their authentic lives.

MORAL CERTAINTY
An Article by SlaveMaster

Another dead-end in life is trying to understand moral certainty before it has been experienced. Trying to make comparisons to other human reactions is misleading and can prevent our doing what must be done to find moral certainty. There are no short cuts, and understanding is a deep hole where no light is shed on the process.

Moral Certainty is an order, and not a feeling at all. There is no appearance of being either right, wrong, good or bad, since those are egotistic conclusions of morality. Moral certainty is not related to having epiphanies, insight or enlightenment. And, certainly, how it "appears" to us or others has no relevance at all.

Moral certainty is a sense of knowing "This must be done!" without logic, without understanding, without reason, and without any supportive feeling. We might actually feel bad about it, because it is the ego which is feeling, not the spirit. Moral certainty doesn't care how we feel, nor does it inquire. Moral certainty often occurs when what we're doing looks wrong, feels bad, is absurd and illogical, indefensible and eclectic.

To ask what is moral certainty is to have never experienced it. When experienced, moral certainty cannot be confused with or compared to anything else. Moral certainty directs us where all egotistic resources are impotent and ineffective. Moral certainty is a direct implementation of what the Universe wants. There is no concern for what we want included. What we want is useful only during the part of life that prepares us for moral certainty.

What's sad is that all the common egotistic rhetoric is what prevents our search for a replacement to reason. What I can guarantee is that happiness will never be found in the mind's rhetoric. The whole point of Born slavery is that it is spiritual, and it will not and cannot follow the psychological, religious or logical tenets of life. What is authentic is a replacement, not a clever combination of all these things.

Growth occurs only when we incorporate and integrate our experiences, not when we discuss our understandings. I've often referred to "understanding" as being like the sound of swirling marbles in a can. Those swirling marbles serve the same purpose and have the same value in our lives as understanding. If the mind could reason to the "Truth," we wouldn't need to live our lives at all. We could put some "roots" on our brains for nutrition and spend our lifetime merely thinking. We are more than our brains, and aren't our brains at all!

What guides us in life has nothing to do with Truth. Does a violinist play violin because it is True? Does a conductor pick music based on its Truth? Yet, each is drawn to do in life what s/he needs because of the draw the instrument or the sound has, and that leads to useful experience.

Without logic, without understanding and without the egotistic test of "Truth," we are led through life, meeting the people we should meet, putting effort into what requires our effort, failing at most things, and succeeding at other things. If it makes "sense," it probably isn't the right thing to do. What the ego thinks is right is what feels safe. The spirit thinks just the opposite.

Obedience is a blank check written against upcoming experience. When our lives are full of blank checks, each will be filled out with moral certainty. Until then, we are only listening to marbles swirling in a can, the noise our egos make inside our heads.

Ignore the noise, and we'll have the time and opportunity to practice issuing our blank checks of obedience, whether Master or slave. When we have a blank check waiting at all times, we will each be granted moral certainty. Until then, everything is doubtful. Everything is uncertain. Everything is unknown. Everything is confusing. That's the way it is supposed to be. Know that, and we'll each outgrow this long phase. Resist it with futile attempts to understand, and we're doomed to stay in the same place.

When we finally accept that our ego IS the enemy, we are free to look for the real solutions that can come only from experience. If we have to be sure, have everything understood and guaranteed in advance, and are not willing to make the necessary mistakes, then the real solutions will never come. Our unwavering search for obedience is the core of authenticity that our honest pursuit will ultimately yield.

If our life pursuits don't build obedience, then we're not getting any closer to moral certainty. Remain confused as long as we must to accept the alternative of obedience, but recognize that it is a diversion and a distraction, not a solution. When we quit trying to understand, then confusion will automatically disappear. It's only our fervent lock on the need to understand that assures confusion.

I know that each of us has to try to prove there is another way. None of us is exempt. Our purpose here is to support each other while we go through the needed dead-end paths that will ultimately convince us that obedience without understanding is the only way to find moral certainty. Moral certainty is worth finding.

It is best for us to develop a humorous sense of acceptance of all the silly things we have to go through while we become more comfortable with not understanding what cannot be understood. We must give up on rooting our brains in one place while we figure this all out in our heads. Invite every experience, and allow others to help put those experiences into perspective to get the most out of each experience.

Let's enjoy it together.

WHAT'S IN A NAME?
An Article by SlaveMaster

Whether a slave, a faggot, a bitch, no matter what the name, it must make no difference. Arrogance is the bane of slavery, of slave development and of spiritual evolution.

Some need a politically incorrect title to feel authentically in the right place to accept who they are, and to accept the obedience which inevitably gives their life its unique purpose and meaning. Being politically correct and being spiritual can be at odds in the world of authenticity and growth.

Having the courage to accept who we are includes having the courage to give up the easy titles that apply previous respect and responsibilities to who we are. By definition, destiny is unique. Using someone else's title, having a place through belonging that comes from association with others of the same title, is not unique. Belonging isn't wrong, belonging simply isn't the process that empowers our unique destiny.

Some see their progression as being one of "boy," to "slave," and then to "Master." Others feel the need to go from faggot, to son, to soldier. Some want only to be one thing, a "slave." What is important is that the title NOT be entitling.

Any egotistic arrogance that either desires or resists any particular title will prevent the open mentality required for growth. Each of our lives is about obedience. Who or what we obey is the biggest single decision we make in life, and it may be the only real human choice we make in life which isn't simply the product of the human machinery made of genetics, conditioning, education and a variety of experiences that define us humanly.

Spiritual evolution through S/M is both authentic and unique as a methodology to growing into who we really are in the larger scheme of things. Growth through S/M includes a "giver," someone who carries the intention of that growth. When combined with the consent of someone willing to accept the product of that intention, there is nothing on earth which matches the focus and intensity of such a practice, for those of us for whom it is natural.

It isn't necessary to tell anyone whether or not S/M as a spiritual practice is natural for them. I'm pretty sure that My mother is not a candidate, and am equally as convinced there are those for whom it is the only effective spiritual practice. You know who you are.

The mind must be prepared, and it must be in the right place to invite the experience of spiritual growth. Consent is part of that preparation. Another part is the availability of its identity.

When a special Someone agrees to take the necessary responsibility to hold the proper intentions to provide growth, they need access to the most vulnerable parts of the ego. How we think of ourselves, the titles by which we are known, is obviously one of the most vulnerable.

The title by which we advertise ourselves, online and in person, can be meant to invite others to accept us and treat us in ways that capture our heart and spirit to fulfill the instinctive need inside. The less we think we are, the more quickly we may become valuable in responsible hands. The danger is in being treated abusively because our value isn't recognized and accepted simultaneously with our lack of egotistic worth that the title would imply.

Sometimes the assigned title needs to change dynamically to match the moment. Whoever holds the agenda must be true to him- or herself in the moment to be effective. Freedom to call the developing spirit by whatever name comes to mind in the moment can maintain an authentic consistency that is otherwise lost.

Words can be powerful. Being associated in one moment with a demeaning, degrading title, and then in the next moment with a different title that is universally powerful can communicate and establish the feeling needed at the time to match some coincidental action that is being taken to form the evolutionary experience.

To desire a name or resist a title makes the ego too active to tolerate growth. Limiting growth is, of course, the whole point of the ego. For those who still entertain the illusion of control, to grow is to change, and the only purpose of control is to retard the rate of change, holding it at zero if possible.

S/M and spiritual growth is the practical implementation of the dynamics of obedience. Self-esteem is exclusively a function of the quality of obedience, and any other measure of self-esteem is egotistic and therefore detrimental to growth. As detrimental to growth as it is, artificially perpetuating the illusion of control is a powerful egotistic agenda despite its fatal effect on real growth.

The willingness to be called by any name can be used as a test of the condition of the ego. A healthy ego, even though valuable in early spiritual development, is an absolute barrier to the later development that yields personal destiny.

What name do you deserve to be called?

Additional Thoughts on Names

slave 7:

"Faggot" brings up all sorts of connotations for people, so using it at large isn't going to end the need to negotiate the meanings of terms over and over again. But, in terms of the gay male slave, "faggot" actually works quite well. The term doesn't lend itself to ego misuse. It is hard to see "faggot" as ever coming to mean King or Lord. And faggot seems to denote the 'gay' male slave's preoccupation with lusting after the male physique. For SlaveMaster and some of His slaves, "faggot" seems to denote some sort of creature that is not quite the same as human, and none of the homophobic uses and connotations the term faggot brings up in society seem to be present when SlaveMaster uses the term, or when many slaves use the term. In short, there doesn't seem to be a term in existence that truly states what this slave is, and SlaveMaster and others often prefer "faggot" over "slave."

OBEDIENCE

An Article by SlaveMaster

It is the heart, character and fiber of a slave to be obedient. Obedience is the prompt, eager and cheerful wanting only what its Owner wants. It is disobedient for a slave to:

Indulge in, express, display or act out anger, moodiness, or any form of disruptive emotion, behavior, or thought. Such characteristics are a violation of cheerfulness.

Display by tone, body language or expression its disagreement with, evaluation of or lack of earnest acceptance of any order. It is a violation of eagerness to do so.

Delay beginning any action. The "Sir, Yes Sir. Thank You, Sir!" which follows any order is expressed while the action begins. Any sign of stall, diversion, creation of extra movements or behavior is a violation of promptness.

Judge or criticize anyone or anything. This is an arrogant, destructive and disobedient activity that isn't tolerated because of its adversity to, and inconsistency with, the character of a slave.

Gossip about another slave, a Master, the SlaveMaster, or any other person, no matter how cleverly disguised by the ego as "discussion." It is a negative activity that involves judgment and prevents slavery. Slaves are encouraged to discuss themselves, their own reactions, and to talk with and about those who are present in the conversation whenever they are otherwise free to be in conversation.

Complain about anything or anyone. A slave is invited to discuss anything with its SlaveMaster. With anyone else, no complaint whatsoever shall ever be expressed by word, action, tone, body language or other means. Complaints are nothing but a poorly-disguised form of excuse. Excuses prevent change. Without change, growth is impossible.

There is obedience and there is *obedience*. What is commonly referred to as obedience is compliance to orders. What slaves require is an alignment of the will so complete that execution can occur without an order being expressed and so immediate the reaction is spontaneous.

Compliance goes through the mind. Obedience doesn't. The work of slave development and related therapy is to rid the slave of all influences and reactions that force each order to go through the head for analysis before being acted upon.

Any issue of trust, self-esteem, self-image, fear, doubts, weakness, bad habits, need for justice, dishonesty, or any other conditioned response must be eliminated to instinctively act on real obedience alone. If we have personal doubt about the certainty of being "clean" of these habitual influences, each command must be referred to the mind to determine the legitimacy of the order.

The process of will-alignment begins when we swear to obey unconditionally. Then, any reaction to an order that isn't spontaneous determines exactly where the next slave development work must be done.

Until a slave is powerful enough to offer obedience that is meaningful, an Owner might not be interested. An Owner might consider the slave too undeveloped to accept as slave. If an Owner takes over a slave's life too early, it can actually inhibit the growth necessary to feel powerful.

The reality is that we are going to experience fulfillment only when we, as Owners, are taking our lives seriously in the absolute pursuit of our obedience to a "Source" that cannot be experienced by the five senses, and teaching our slaves that same blind obedience to Us so they can inherit our connection. There are lots of excuses for not doing so. Some of the reasons are based on psychology, and some on the injustice of life's experiences. I could easily list more than a hundred excuses that have been egotistically presented to Me over time.

Obedience can be understood as a connection. That connection can be with others or to something less tangible, but it always makes us a part of what or Who is obeyed.

There is no magic moment in which a slave suddenly feels ready to surrender its obedience completely and without compromise. The magic is only in finding its qualified, destined Owner. When that happens, the question about whether it should obey answers itself. When that happens, every life experience becomes inarguable evidence that it has made the right decision which never again needs to be questioned.

Obedience must be unlimited. Responsibility must be unlimited. No matter what our destinies, the limits we put on our obedience and responsibility are the limits we put on our lives. Everything else is simply the training ground for developing our capacity to obey.

Slaves instinctively know their need to obey. All a slave needs is the opportunity. Giving obedience is all they want to care about, and their spirit yearns to find a place and means to do so. There is no surprise that slaves want to obey. The only surprise would be if they didn't.

Slaves don't prepare for slavery by developing individual skills. Slaves prepare for slavery by developing the ability to really and actually obey. Obedience is wanting and needing only what The Owner gives it to want and need. Nothing else matters and everything else is the egotistic development of the skills résumé useful only for Master/slave negotiation.

Obedience is letting the soul do whatever it wants to do whenever it wants to do it. Don't stand in the way of the soul. Obey It.

Additional Thoughts on Obedience

slave 7:

The slave soul wants and needs to go "home." That is, it needs to join with the Owner soul. And the only way to reunite with the Owner soul is to live in obedience. That is the glue, the connector, the container that holds it all together.

SlaveMaster said, "People keep praying to the Universe and asking for things, but what we need to realize is that the Universe is praying to us... and we need to listen." This struck 7 as a different and beautiful way to look at obedience... that we are merely answering the prayers of the Universe. Disobedience is denying the prayers of the Universe. Our prayers come in the form of worship, thanks and obedience, but it is the Universe that "asks" for things with prayer, not people.

7 chooses obedience in advance. 7 embraces obedience and loves obedience. Obedience brings 7 a feeling of truly

being alive. 7 claims obedience as its right, its joy and its life.

While it may seem extreme or unrealistic to some, obedience and worship are easy for 7, as they both come naturally. If Master and slave are One, then obedience is effortless, for Master and slave are simply in sync. Remember, a slave's obedience is not only to the words of Master, but also to the spirit within and what it calls upon the slave to do, whether Master is physically present or not. Worship helps this slave connect to Master and stay connected, and brings this slave joy.

Perspective

SlaveMaster:

When something isn't true for us now, it doesn't mean it might not be true tomorrow, or after even one more experience which gives us a changed perspective. It is important that we encourage each other to express exactly what each feels and to invite radically-varying opinions in response. This is the objective and the process by which we can see where we have been, where we are now, and where we might be going. To a child, a parent leaving it with a baby sitter to go to the store can look like abandonment. As the beliefs change through experience that same child will eventually recognize the gift of the parent leaving to acquire what it needs. The action is the same, but the understanding and perspective change.

Protocol

SlaveMaster:

Use whatever protocol works for you, but accept the limit and position that slaves fully meant to be slaves are put in by doing so. No action is without consequences. Limit the framework within which a slave lives and grows, and the strength and freedom of the slave contained by that framework is limited.

slave 7:

Compliance to SlaveMaster's protocol is not in itself obedience. It is merely compliance. It provides the slave the environment in which obedience can gain a foothold and then grow. The protocol is a living, never-stopping meditation and a way for the slave to focus on Master, as well as inner being, which is also part of Master. In this never-ending meditation, old distractions are not allowed entry and the slave begins to notice life anew. A new 'voice' is heard; a new centeredness is attained. When the slave begins to follow the newly-identified voice, obedience begins. When the slave naturally and habitually and spontaneously lives by this voice, then obedience is reached and slavery begins. Add worship of Master to this, and you have a properly focused, obedient slave.

Protocol has real purpose: it provides the environment in which a slave can find its self (or inner voice), grow, and learn obedience. Protocol works more productively when the slave actively embraces it and lives it. Protocol can work while the Master is not physically present. It is not static; it may change and grow to best suit where the slave is in its development (and development is never-ending). Routine and ritual only have effect when applied and embraced according to the need at hand.

Punishment

slave 7:

Many slaves, including this one to some degree, have had some sort of fantasy about being punished. It feels nice to know that Master has the power and right to punish, but having lived real time as slave to SlaveMaster this slave has come to realize the power of being slave without any threat (or hope) of punishment. It seems to this slave that punishment may limit the depth of slavery attained by allowing the slave to possibly have the sense of only being slave (and therefore obedient) due to threat of punishment, taking away a sense in the slave that it obeys because it IS slave, because that is what it does, by self-recognition and self-acceptance only. In short, punishment may limit the full realization of the slave self by allowing the ego a foothold.

SlaveMaster disciplines, providing what a slave needs in order to let the slave self out to live in full. How can a slave live without self-control and self-interest if there is not a Master/Owner to take over that control and interest? SlaveMaster gladly takes over the control and interest of the slave, not with punishment, but with discipline. The slave merely needs be true to itself, and it will have no need for punishment.

A Born slave must recognize its spiritual reality and live its life accordingly, void of the need for punishment, fully obedient only because it IS its Owner's slave.

SlaveMaster does not punish a slave for not living up to protocol with 100% success. In fact, SlaveMaster NEVER punishes. Never. He believes that punishment will not lead to success. Rather, slaves learn to give, from the heart, with no help or threat of punishment. Protocol, routine and discipline enable and empower a slave so that it may embrace its calling.

Success for a Born slave comes from one's acceptance of that calling, not from any enforcement from a Master. If SlaveMaster's hand doesn't do what He wants it to do, He doesn't punish His hand. Rather, He looks for the causes of the problem and seeks to rectify those.

WHEN TO QUIT
An Article by SlaveMaster

If you don't feel your slavery, and it isn't something that you want to pursue any longer, then it is appropriate to remove the collar, go another direction, for now or forever.

When a person is developing who they really are, in obedience to another, there isn't anything, any circumstance, about that which makes me uncomfortable. What others carp about isn't any of my concern at all. I do only what is in integrity for me. The results are what they are. I don't adjust my protocol, my life or my concerns to accommodate anyone.

The only question that is pertinent is whether or not you can be in integrity with the life that you're living. No other concern is relevant.

Born slavery is self-defined, and I am only its witness. I don't control its parameters, and don't adjust its members. The point is to have a life of helping others. The "others" will take on many forms. Slavery that isn't based on pure, uncompromised honesty and the pursuit of destiny isn't slavery at all. Others misuse of the word doesn't change what slavery is.

Anyone who retains the right to not be honest, or to control where their life will go is egotistic, and not pursuing destiny. Egotism and destiny are mutually exclusive. Destiny is a high calling, and it demands everything we are and think.

It's okay to be pursuing destiny, or not to be. Each type of person needs assistance and support, and each can give assistance and support to others.

Truth learned through any experience is worth knowing, and makes the experience worthwhile. I have no confusion over whether someone is unabashedly pursuing who they are, or not. The process I witness and am a part of is of that unabashed pursuit.

I will never be concerned about what makes others uncomfortable or causes them to "carp." It is my job to, in fact, expose people to what makes them uncomfortable or makes them carp, not by intention, but from telling the truth. That's what forces growth and development. When we stay within the same comfort zone, then nothing changes, and without change there is no growth.

Everyone knows what they are willing to do for or give to any process. Everyone knows what they are willing to invest in their pursuits. Everyone knows how far out of their comfort zone they are willing to move or live. I accept those limits. I precisely define what it does take so others will know what the cost of having integrity is. Each has to weigh that cost against the benefits, and the importance of those benefits to themselves.

The only question is what you want to do. Whatever that is, is fine. You have to feel your own integrity. But it's not about others' confusion, or what others feel, think or do.

Usually, when you've asked the question about continuing with your slavery, you've already made a decision, you've already made up your mind, and that's okay. It takes as much courage to find out what doesn't work for us, what doesn't fulfill our lives, as it does to pursue that which does. Do what your doubts tell you to do, and don't look back!

WHEN IS A SLAVE READY?
An Article by SlaveMaster

The process of becoming slave requires several things, including:

- Learning complete obedience

- Acceptance of who you are, no matter what that is

- Doing with your life whatever, whoever, whenever you are ordered, forever

- Giving up all claim to a self

- Growing in the perfect, fertile environment for a slave

- Being part of a family of slaves

- Allowing yourself to experience that there is a higher power that will run your life

The person who does the developing has to:

- Have as his sole objective first the development, then Be the one who was given who you are management, of your slavery

- Be internally sworn to always act in the slave's best interest, for life

- Know how to give slavery

- Have accepted his own destiny, and be following the Universe's orders, intentionally

If any of the above elements is missing, then you are arranging a relationship, not pursuing your destiny as a slave. Either process is legitimate, but different. If you were given your own purpose, you should arrange your own relationships. If your purpose was given to another, you should never arrange your own relationship.

You either were created to be slave, or you were not.

To decide if you are ready, determine:

- Whether or not you were given your own purpose or it was given to another.

- If you have developed personally to the point that you are independently successful, and don't need a relationship to "make" you successful.

- If you are willing to give your personal success away for what your creator wants you to do, no matter what that is.

- If slavery is now your first and best choice of what to do in life, not a second or "also- ran" alternative.

- That you have had enough experiences with what doesn't work that you won't go through your slavery development constantly looking over your shoulder at what might be better.

- That you don't have a hidden agenda and are capable of finally wanting ONLY what another wants for the rest of your life.

- If you have the commitment, perseverance and dedication to do whatever is required to first become, and then live your slavery.

- If you will let yourself become proud of your slavery, first to yourself, then others, and then to the world.

- If you are willing to accept the responsibility of being a leader in life, and of doing what it requires to be great, in obedience.

- If you are willing to accept being a non-human creature incapable of committing an immoral act, ever, for the rest of your life.

Becoming slave is not a battle of the wills or of the egos. It is accepting that the only will you have or want is your owner's will, and there is only one will.

Before beginning, REVIEW:

- Personally and privately where you currently are in light of the above requirements

- With friends, potential slave brothers, family and others whose opinion you respect

- With the man or woman you think was created with your purpose

Only then is it time to arrange the first session. In most cases you will know after the first session whether or not you are slave, or have the ability to become what you were created to be. You also have to be willing to accept the truth about that.

Additional Thoughts on Readiness

slave 7:

7 discovered some funny things about doors: They can be right in front of you and you may not even see them. If you open one, then you wind up in a room with more doors. You can easily refuse to open a door. You can open a door just a crack, take a small peek, and then close it and pretend you saw nothing. You can demand to know what is behind a door and where it leads before opening it and entering. But you will never know until you open the door and step through. You can open a door before you are ready for what lies beyond it. So, there are times when keeping a door closed until a later point in life is necessary. The door you yearn for may be very far off and out of reach, for now. You can't predict where a door may lead, or choose a path to where you think you want to go. Doors just lead to wherever they lead. Doors can lead to things you never thought possible. Doors do not close behind you, at least not to the extent that you don't know where you came from. You may never know where a door is going to be. Only you have your doors. They are especially for you and no one else. There is darkness and light behind doors. Doors can be easy to open or difficult to open. And a door can just open up for you when you are near it. Sometimes, you step through doors you didn't even see until after the fact. Somewhere inside you is a quality (a heart, spirit, soul?) that draws you toward your doors. You can choose to listen to that quality, or you can choose to ignore it.

This slave does, on occasion, meet unowned slaves who have desired slavery for most of their lives and have come to believe that an Owner does not exist. Years ago, when this slave came to truly accept that no Owner exists, and was completely fine with that, finally at peace, no longer caring that an Owner does not exist, totally accepting what life brought—even the lack of slavery—Master arrived, for the slave was ready.

When a slave loses its desperation for a Master, such slave may actually be ready for its Master. Indifference, not desperation, indicates one's readiness to obey.

When thinking about readiness for slavery, consider whether you are ready to have someone refine your diet to meet certain health standards, or whether you are ready to let someone tell you how to brush your teeth for optimal oral hygiene, or how to drive properly. BDSM is the least of your worries. More slaves have been chased away by SlaveMaster's order to not drink diet soda than by His flogger.

If the Master is Right, He is worth waiting for. And if the slave is Right, the slave is worth waiting for.

This slave believes that the only connection with another person that is going to 'work,' whether it be a vanilla relationship or a Master-slave, is one in which both parties have not manipulated it in order to try to make it work. We all need to try things that wind up not working, in order to learn, grow, and find out what is right for us.

Expect what is natural, and it may come. Demand (before something is naturally ready), and a new obstacle is created. Demand, and you have only taken. Expect, and you may receive. Demand as if you Know. Expect as if you Trust.

Religion

SlaveMaster:

Nothing about spiritual evolution, going from spiritual childhood, to adolescence, and then onto adulthood has anything to do with religion. Religion plays a critical part in each of our lives but our spiritual lives are not defined by religion any more than it is defined by our work environment, our family or any other single influence. All of these experiences are how we develop.

slave 7:

While this slave lived life before meeting SlaveMaster, it had the instinctual desire to worship, even though it did not know what to worship. Most often Mother Nature came to mind, but it did not believe in any God, and so it did not worship. It thought about worshiping a Man, but it had no man in its life worthy of worship and did not dream that any man could be worthy of worship, or that worshiping a Man could be an emotionally healthy thing to do. Also, its mind was clouded with definitions and connotations of "worship" that, in the end, don't apply to worship as this slave now understands it. Yes, this slave worships its Owner, SlaveMaster. it bows at His feet and calls Him Master, Great Lord, my Lord, Your Lordship, Beautiful One, Giver of Life, ManGod, Lord and Commander, Controller, Beautiful Man, my Owner, my Source, my Reason for Living, God.

Worship is unlimited giving, unlimited loving, a one way street of all of one's life-energy. it feels cleansing and purifying, as all barriers, limitations, hesitations, hang ups, are totally burned away. Worship melds one into the Other.

Master as a Whole is worthy of worship, as are each of His body parts. Anything connected with Master is worthy of worship. During acts of worship, every fiber of this slave animal comes to life, with an erection, with joy, with the vibrant thrill of being alive... with flowing INTO its Master and leaving separateness behind.

Resistance

slave 7:

7 is different from most who begin actual slave development in that it had little resistance, but that is because this slave had known it is slave for virtually all of its adult life and had come to terms with it. Life before its slavery absolutely sucked, so there was nothing to give up, and once it met SlaveMaster, it simply knew it was in the right place, with the right Owner, so there was no reason to resist.

This slave did have plenty of resistance when it met up with Masters whom it felt were not the One. it knew internally (without really even thinking about it) that it simply wasn't the right time for its slavery to begin.

If you are a Born slave, you are not "another," as in an individual soul, but "of another," as in one part of a larger soul (or all the Universe) that inhabits more than one body. But, of course, don't take 7's word for it. Find out for yourself! Seriously. There is certainly nothing wrong with, and still every reason to be, "self" protective and resistant. Being careful is a good thing.

A slave doesn't feel alone unless it actively rejects its Owner. And if a slave rejects its Owner, it rejects its Self.

Many resist their own calling to be slave due to a strong need to be independent men, self-responsible, free of dependence on a another Man to direct them. Horseshit.

Rights

slave 7:

But the slave owns the right to obey. The right to obey is the totality of life for a slave and everything a slave needs. The right to obey and obedience are all-inclusive. No other right need exist. Rights like "the right not to be abused" is covered under Master's responsibility to take care of His slave and do what is in its best interest, and the right is the SlaveMaster's right, and the SlaveMaster's responsibility, and He fends for it... and obedience fends for it.

A slave doesn't have any rights because a slave doesn't need any rights. The SlaveMaster takes all the rights as His own. He takes all the responsibility, and gives the slave all the freedom to obey its spirit.

When slaves speak of having rights, they are normally referring to having a way to protect themselves from their Masters. If a slave needs to be concerned about such rights with a Master, then that may be a good sign that the Master is not Right.

Searching

slave 7:

So, in what state of being do you feel most alive? Or, what elements give you the sense that you are alive, grounded, and real? It seems to this slave that that is the search. When and if one finally feels the "rapture of being alive" just from being in the here and now, being fully present and centered, as the jargon goes, and purified of the life influences that get thrown upon us since Day 1, one may have a mental construct of what constitutes reality, but one may also know that that construct means little and matters little. Knowing your own little piece of it is all that matters. One piece of a puzzle need only fit into the next. it doesn't need to know how the whole puzzle fits together, or how it operates, or if it is the only puzzle.

Self-Acceptance

slave 7:

This slave became independent when it became slave. Independent of bullshit, oppressive norms, independent of what others think of "me," and independent from what "I" think of me. Purely independent, being exactly what i am, as i am... free to be as is. This slave became independent when it became slave.

Sexual Service

SlaveMaster:

We are beyond seeing slavery as something a person does to deliver sex to someone who cares for them financially and emotionally in exchange. The slave-fantasy dream of being used sexually in exchange for complete security, and the Master-fantasy of having someone to provide any manner of sexual service in exchange for providing all of life's other needs, always ends in frustration. That doesn't stop any of us, however, from thinking we'll be the first to be successful. That's how the ego works.

slave 7:

Yes, those things between your legs are Master's, not yours to play with nor think about. All you have to do is dive into your Master and live there. He, nature and the Universe take care of the rest.

Chastity doesn't lead to a lack of eroticism; it leads to more. It collects the energy and empowers the slave. It leads the slave to become a passionate, drooling animal intent on crawling to and into Him. It brings the slave to life.

The core elements of this slave's sex drive, from its earliest memories of feeling it, are about being slave to a Man. Not having sex with a Man, but being connected to a Man as His slave, which involves sex acts, but also a great eroticism around things that are not sex acts at all, like simply being a dog or horse, or kneeling before Him, or just being at His feet while He looks at it knowingly. its lifelong biggest turn-on is not even a physical act, but the thought of being OWNED.

One giant change for this slave once it met SlaveMaster was that for the first time in its life it could remain present in the moment during erotic acts. Before being with SlaveMaster, it usually had to fantasize about slave-things that were not actually happening in order to stay aroused. Now, just being with Master, being totally present, just being slave, just BEING, is arousing.

This slave encounters over and over again, as it did in the media and among people in general, prior to ever self-actualizing as slave, the perception that a gay male slave is a sex toy and lives in a cage all day. Perhaps it is true in some quarters, but certainly not in Born slavery. Born slavery is not about sex. It is about being one's purest self, and understanding that self as a tool, not a toy, for a greater good.

slave 7 defines his greatest fetish as being SlaveSexual:

SlaveSexual: (adj.): sexually attracted to, or erotically charged by, elements of personal slavery more so than by sexual acts; aroused by actualities and concepts such as:

- Belonging to someone

- Giving up control

- Being used as a servant

- Being held in intimate bondage

- Being connected to another

- Being expected to worship in unrestrained love

- Being as free as an animal

- Living without mental-emotional boundaries

- Having a sense of purpose in servitude and betterment of life for others

- Feeling the support and acceptance of an Owner who, via ownership of them, enables one's life forces within

- Being at one with nature, feeling a part of nature

- Feeling separate from humanity for the purpose of serving humanity

A SLAVE OR SERVANT?

An Article by slave 7

Some use the term Master and some use the term Owner. Here, these terms are used interchangeably. These thoughts are about a slave, and are from a slave's perspective.

Slavery is about having no options, about being totally owned and operated. A slave is not a free man who has decided to grant services to a Master. A slave does not even seek to please a Master. Seeking to please is a concern of the ego. Seeking to please is just one more way for the ego to say, "See! I'm good!" But a slave feels no such concerns. A slave understands that the ego is what stands in the way of true slavery and of the authentic connection to the Master or Owner. The ego is the enemy of slavery, so seeking to please a Master automatically destroys slavery.

Any slave granting a Master services rather than obeying is a servant, not a slave. Slaves do not grant services, they obey. Any Master who has found a man who "slaves" for him, who calls him "Master" and runs around serving him all day, is not a Master, but merely a recipient of voluntary services. Masters do not simply receive, they give commands.

A slave seeks only one thing: obedience, to be trapped into obedience so that no sense of choice clouds its heart, mind and spirit, an obedience so strong that the slave IS obedience, and that the slave becomes One with the Owner, an intimacy so great and powerful that no other pleasure in life need exist.

Some may suggest that being so obedient means being mindless, but this is not the case. Obedience means having no selfish thoughts of one's own, while listening with ears, heart and spirit for any order given.

Any order given may require that the slave make great use of mental powers, although they are used in obedience rather than to achieve the objectives of the ego.

Just obey, and authentic slavery follows. Just serve, and there is no slavery because no one is Master.

Additional Thoughts on Service

slave 7:

It is not really true that a slave works without reward. There are many rewards, but they are the rewards that the Universe grants when one lives authentically and true to spirit and destiny. What seems important is that one not have any sense of tit-for-tat for service, no "if i do this, then i'll get that." Those are ego-determined rewards. In this slave's experience, the greatest rewards are ones we can't foresee, and they come from a place other than where we are looking. They are not linked to specific acts of service. They do not come as rewards for any such acts. Born slavery itself is a reward, an honor, a joy... and easy... if one is designed to be this type of slave.

Service can be an act of the ego and, therefore, is subject to flaws. Obedience is an act of heart and spirit, and, therefore, is not subject to flaws. A Born slave is of service only through obedience. This slave sees service as a conscious act, a considered act, a decision and motivation of the ego, and therefore very likely to be contaminated with personal agenda and perspective.

Genuine service occurs naturally when one obeys. Service is merely an offshoot of obedience. Problems arise, though, because the mind (ego) has a set of rules for what service is and must look like, and the Orders of the heart and spirit do not fit into that set of rules. In fact, what one feels is the right thing to do in the heart (an Order) may look completely contrary to what the mind believes is service. The point is: allow the heart to override the ego idea of service and proceed with continued obedience and listening within. This is exactly the point of obedience.

The ego doesn't know what kind of service is needed, or whom exactly to serve.

We act in obedience and don't even know who benefits or how. We may never know how we serve. We just have faith that we are serving the will of the Universe because we are listening to the authentic, divine voice. In serving the will of the Universe, we are serving and doing right by others. What seems unkind or even a disservice to some human eyes may be the perfect service to the will of the universe. We may see a situation in which service is needed, and yet the best service we can render is to not become involved, because the Universe has willed something we don't know about nor need to know about. We only know that ours is not to become involved. What service to provide is different for everyone. This is part of what makes each one of us unique. We are all uniquely qualified to serve unique people in unique circumstances. We serve just by being our true selves.

SlaveMaster defines "service" far differently than most Masters. He doesn't define it as any direct action toward or for his personal Being. Just being one's authentic self is service to SlaveMaster.

Soul

SlaveMaster:
Accepting that the soul owns us makes it a lot easier to say "yes" to the destiny question about acting for the Creator's purpose instead of our own. Happiness, from the vantage point that the soul owns us, isn't any more demanding than letting the soul do whatever it wants to do

whenever it wants to do it. Happiness becomes a function of simply not standing in the way of the soul, objecting to its desires and functions. Our challenge is to learn how to let go and let the soul do its work. It is the only challenge that matters in the bigger scheme of things. Everything else is merely preparation for that.

The soul owns us. That acceptance will give us the courage to let the soul experience what it wants to experience. Take a quiet moment. Examine your life in light of the soul owning you. Witness how much more sense everything that has happened in your life makes. Consider how much less it looks like we're risking when we view the soul as being the possessor instead of our possession.

WHAT IS THE SPIRIT OF A SLAVE?
An Article by SlaveMaster

Who a slave is was given to another by the slave's Creator. This is the only difference between a slave and any other man or woman who accepts the destiny for which each was designed. Let's explore how that feels to a potential slave, and how a slave might recognize whether or not the slave spirit is present.

There is a special spirit inside every slave. That spirit is unique in all the world but holds common characteristics with all others who are created to be slave. It was placed there before conception by the Creator in accordance with the agreement reached with the soul. The slave spirit is a very natural, unaffected animal, very much like the other animals of the world. Interchangeably, the words slave, spirit and animal can be used once the real nature of slavery is understood.

They all make reference to the same entity within anyone who is slave.

Why is it so difficult to accept being a slave?

The challenge is in the ego. Our whole life we are taught that we are who we are referring to when we say "I" or "me." Everyone in our support system convinces us the ego reference is to who we are. Everything we encounter while growing up refers to our need to identify and develop everything that we egotistically discover, are consciously aware of, and think that we want.

While we are each occupied with the process of taking care of our personal development, the slave animal remains dormant. The spirit patiently awaits a suitable environment into which it can come to life. The spirit is wise, and always has been. It won't expose itself to anything that isn't in its best interest and that doesn't contribute to its well-being. If the necessary conditions are never encountered, the slave will never take its first breath. Those conditions are demanding. They must support a destined life.

At times during a slave's development, either consciously or by accident, there are temporary situations which will evoke a response from the animal. It will expose itself for a brief and controlled amount of time. The experience confirms to us the existence of the spirit, and encourages us to continue the pursuit of slavery. These glimpses into who we really are, along with the appetites we usually call fetishes, encourage us to explore further.

What the spirit really searches for, however, is an environment in which it can come to life, grow and never have to return to its dormant state. It is the spirit's purpose to locate and accept the environment in which that can be done.

What does it take for the slave to find the environment it needs?

The slave's limitation is that it can never produce its own environment. The spirit requires its owner, the one who shares its spirit. Only the owner can direct that part of himself, the slave part, and empower the necessary growth. That is the challenge of slavery.

Slavery isn't about relationships, activities, protocols or titles. Slavery is about the search for, and acceptance of, the Owner who can give the spirit the opportunity to live. The Creator who placed the spirit inside doesn't give someone a destiny of slavery and then not provide the opportunity for it to develop. The egotistic human who contains the spirit doesn't perform the search for an owner, the spirit itself finds and presents the owner when the spirit is ready.

The struggle is with time. The spirit can't and won't accept its destiny until it is completely ready. And, until it is ready, there is nothing the egotistic slave can do to accelerate the process. When the spirit is prepared, the Creator will provide the "coincidence" necessary for its development to begin. The slave doesn't have to arrange for it. The slave has to be open to it.

The egotistic slave doesn't even know when he's ready, but the spirit does. Therefore, it is the slave's job to accept the opportunity to come to life when it is presented, not to create the opportunity in the first place.

The slave gets confused along the way. There is this long period of time between when we are born and when we are prepared to accept our destiny. During that time, our S/M and other appetites direct the search to experiences which yield temporary satisfaction. These experiences are quick looks at the way it could and should be. A danger is presented during the wait. When these partial, temporary experiences feel beneficial, the slave can be lulled into thinking it is his job to make the temporary experience permanent.

There is nothing instinctive that tells a slave that his experiences are intended to prepare him for his destiny, not to be the fulfillment of it. There is nothing in the slave's instincts which tell him that his job is to accept someone else as his owner. The slave usually feels his connection through a need to provide service, not find the single owner of the spirit that lives inside. The slave concludes that it is his job to find a relationship, instead of his destiny.

As more egotistic success is achieved, the slave continues to explore the same type of negotiated arrangements that yielded initial temporary benefits. This process is much like enjoying our sophomore year, and working at repeating it over and over for a lifetime. Frustration is the result. The ego, and the intellect with which we support the ego, make the process even more difficult.

Personal development has as its objective becoming egotistically strong. Being egotistically developed is what prepares us to accept our destiny. In fact, it is critical to the process of becoming egotistically successful. The ego, however, concludes that personal development is the same as destiny. So, it believes, being completely egotistic is the fulfillment of who we are.

Until a slave knows better, it is the inevitable belief that he is who his ego is. Our society, our therapists, our friends and our families all confirm our erroneous belief. There are few clues that we should even be looking into someone else to find who we are. We settle for the popular thought: our egos are who we are.

Only the one nagging feeling that something is still missing causes us to question the error of our conclusion about the ego. It takes courage and strength to look for an answer in places that everyone is telling us it is crazy to look. There is no support system for encouraging anyone to explore slavery as the answer to their spiritual aspirations. Finding who we are in someone else sounds too much like co-dependence and we've spent a fortune getting over that. Being a slave sounds too much like what we fought a civil war for, and for what many have died for to have the freedom to be who they were meant to be.

Slavery is neither co-dependence nor the imposed submission that others have suffered throughout history. The ego intentionally misunderstands the difference as an excuse not to walk the path for which a slave was created. So long as the ego can argue that there is no solution, it doesn't have to accept one.

So, what happens then?

Life's experiences challenge the slave to let go. The slave begins to feel afraid. Egotistically, our training and development have taught us that we need to "take control," become personally directed, set our own goals, make things happen for ourselves and create our own reality.

Letting go threatens all of the egotistic achievements that have been a sign of our success. Letting go taps into the fear of not being able to control our life, not being able to self-control our dark nature which might want to do something wrong. Or, it might want to do something that others wouldn't approve of. We know we would lose our right to negotiate for anything if we let go. We "enjoy" the fear of not being able to pursue what we want.

Our success at negotiating for a successful weekend, or week, or month, or six months, leads the slave to feel that all he needs is the right to negotiate the same thing for a life time. That's not how life works. That's not how the spirit works. That's not how relationships work.

The spirit must be let go; it must be set free. Like any animal, all spirits need the adventure of discovery to find out who they are. Kept in a cage the size of the body, no one will ever learn the nature of what is caged. Self-control is a self-made prison the same size as the body. The perfectionist takes pride in how small the prison is. The perfectionist's height of achievement is building a space so small that there isn't room to make a mistake.

In real life, in authentic slaves, the result of our self-made prison is that the spirit never comes to life because of the limited size of its containment. It doesn't even try to live. It has the wisdom not to try to grow in an environment that won't support it.

How, then, can the spirit be allowed to live?

The slave spirit must be controlled by another. It cannot live when it has any right to negotiate. It has no life so long as it can want for itself. It can feel only fear until it can find someone to whom it can give unqualified obedience.

To whom can a slave give unqualified obedience?

The spirit must find its owner. That is very different from finding the human body's owner. This distinction is where the misunderstanding of property, and of rights has come from. Egotistic slaves still think they have the right to negotiate for the owner of their body, while they retain their own egotistic control of the spirit.

The spirit owns the body, not the ego. The owner owns the spirit, and in the same way as he owns his own spirit. It is owned not as property, but as self-identification. When the body is owned directly, then it is merely property. That denigrates and denies the value of a slave. A slave cannot be property. That would be to have less value, and less protection than provided

163

by the S.P.C.A. and laws that protect animals. There is nothing lesser about a slave. A slave is destined.

The egotistic objection to not using "I" and "me" is a reflection of the fear and reluctance to admit that the ego doesn't own who a slave is. To acknowledge that the slave spirit owns the body is to acknowledge the ego has no rights, has no control over who the slave is, nor over what it does, nor with whom it has a connection.

When it isn't clear that the soul — the slave spirit — owns the body, the whole point of slavery is missed. Missing the whole point is the purpose of the ego. To indulge the ego is to continue to miss the point, the purpose, and the solutions to a slave's fulfillment and happiness.

How does the slave spirit grow?

It first has to grow through the egotistic preparation for its destiny. For someone who is slave, the chronic egotistic control of the internal spirit eventually feels like an overwhelming burden. It doesn't feel right to a slave to always have to exercise egotistic control. The natural appetites of a slave for S/M power, and the security of bondage, plus all the other instinctive appetites drive the slave spirit to seek and explore.

Some who are slave — some who have always carried the spirit inside — willingly submit to S/M as an egotistically-controlled release for the agreed-to amount of time that will allow the spirit to feel some freedom. Afterwards, the spirit is put back to sleep by the re-emergence of the ego's self-control. This allows the slave to be controllably out of control. The spirit can be temporarily released without actually giving it any power over, or any control of the "real" parts of life.

The appetites remain unrequited, regardless of what diversions and distractions are performed, so long as the ego has any rights or influence. The ego feels it must stay powerful to prevent the spirit from running wild. The ego is convinced that without itself we would follow the spirit and do unreasonable, unthinkable, embarrassing, disgusting things that others would criticize. We fear being thought of as having "unseemly exuberance."

The spirit is always experienced as being powerful and playful. There is a natural fear of giving anything that is so powerful and uncontrollable its "head," because it could do things that are not controlled and that might expose the slave. This brings out another fear that is similar to the feeling of being outed. It feels like arranging for our own self-outing, by a part of ourselves that we can't keep under control. It is no wonder that we find such clever and relentless egotistic objections to putting ourselves into a position where we could expose ourselves to such behavior and results.

A slave, therefore, simultaneously feels that it wants to be controlled by another and at the same time needs to egotistically remain in control to insure an environment that makes sense, that is reasonable, and that doesn't denigrate the value or esteem of the slave. This is a dilemma. How can you act like a slave and still remain in a position powerful enough to assure protection of the slave's well-being and best interest?

What is the solution?

Two conditions must be present. First, the slave's ego must be powerless so that there is no one but the owner to control the owner's spirit inside the slave. Second, the owner must act with a responsibility for the slave that is superior to the slave's potential or actualized responsibility for himself.

Why would anyone be motivated to take on such a responsibility?

Only someone who truly and absolutely considers the slave to be a part of himself would be willing. No one would make a life-long commitment to another without believing some immutable connection exists that was created beyond human control, and beyond any human right to dissolve it.

A slave is destined to belong to another. When that other is placed into the slave's life, the spirit is free to grow because, for the first time, there is someone in whom to place the obedience which sets the spirit free.

When is someone ready to begin development?

Each of the Born slaves, and all of those currently committed to the development of their slavery, did not plan on finding an owner. The meeting was both unexpected and compelling. There was no examination, no interview, no research, and no selection process. There was nothing to argue with or against. The spirit insisted, and issued a captivating command. There was no choice, nothing to consider, and nothing logically to discuss. Such meetings are always, and only, the result of a slave's personal prayer of willingness to serve its Creator instead of its own selfish interest.

When someone is still trying to decide whether to accept an owner he isn't ready to begin his slave development. Only after the spirit is prepared can it accept the development of its destiny. Until then, the ego must continue to be developed and matured to ready it to accept the inevitable. Until the ego is developed far enough to know that it has tremendous capacity but still doesn't have any ability to produce happiness, it continues to argue, to consider, to discuss, to explore, to posture and to pretend that it has some control and influence over what must happen, and when it will happen.

The argument and struggle is a confirmation that the ego isn't ready. The spirit is patient, and won't arrange for its development until the willingness that comes from egotistic development is adequate. So long as there remains a conscious doubt, a slave shouldn't consider the development of his slavery because he isn't ready to begin. That doesn't preclude having S/M, bondage, and slavery experiences or relationships. It maturely recognizes that experiences and relationships are different, and therefore not the spiritual development of a slave's destiny. They are, instead, preparation for it.

When the spirit is compelled, because it knows the ego is ready, the opportunity for slave development happens without being arranged through personal effort. It then takes only willingness on the part of the slave. It will probably happen unexpectedly, and when it's NOT something you're looking for. What we egotistically control, the Universe will not fight us for.

When the owner is put into the slave's life, the development of the spirit inside can then start. The spirit has always been a part of its owner. When the owner finds his spirit within a slave, and the slave is willing to give it to its rightful owner, then the conditions are, for the first time, in place for its growth.

What develops the slave spirit?

The slave spirit is too wild, too untamed, and so undomesticated that it cannot be allowed to act on its own until it learns to obey. Common sense has kept it reined in, under self- control, and therefore stifled. The slave cannot begin to know itself until it can explore without self-control. The slave cannot begin to explore until it first learns to obey.

When a slave knows how to obey, and is obeying the only person in whom he can place absolute obedience — the one who will protect the spirit — the slave can finally let go. Life is not about controlling. It is about never being able to control again — never having to, and never wanting to.

The development process is one of exploring to see what the spirit will do, how it will feel, and to find out what it is like. The slave must first learn to know the spirit that lives inside, that has always belonged to another. Then he must learn to trust and love that spirit, because it is all the slave is and will ever be.

The spirit must learn to live and express in the absolutely safe control of the owner through the sessions that both empower and force the spirit to venture into unknown territory. At the same time, it must slowly learn to be allowed to live in obedience for the remainder of life, in the work place, in the family, in school, in hobbies and in every area. It is dipped into complete and safe exposure to experience, then taken out to learn to live in a world when the owner isn't physically present, but is only inside, inside as the spirit that lives within.

The perfectionist will attempt to keep tight egotistic controls on the spirit, to make sure it doesn't do anything wrong. This can keep it from being able to run free at all. There will be a fear of being in any position where control cannot be maintained. Excuses will be found to prevent the opportunity to have a session of exposure. As the willingness to face and accept the truth becomes strong enough, the slave will let the spirit be empowered by its owner, and to let it go anywhere the owner wants it to go.

Only the owner can protect the spirit. Only the owner can empower it to explore. Only the owner can allow the spirit to express itself honestly and without any limits or bounds. The owner forces it into situations, places, and circumstances where it must be exposed. Nothing can or will remain hidden. No agenda nor control will remain undisclosed.

The conscious obedience to the owner is the only lifeline that can allow the spirit to run free. If the owner calls it back from a dangerous place, without obedience, the spirit will continue and run into the potential dangers. When the slave is sure that he will obey, then the spirit can be allowed to go anywhere and everywhere. The owner's knowledge that he has both the ability and the intention of protecting his own spirit inside the slave gives the slave spirit the absolute freedom it must have to grow.

The spirit is forced to go where it can expose the hidden desires for control, or for protection. It is forced to uncover the angers, resentments, disappointments, hatred, blame and judgments that contaminate us. If we control, or feel any response to be inappropriate, then we control all response. We are either open or we are not. We can't be both available and hidden at the same time. Wherever there is any limit, there is every limit.

Honesty is the powerhouse of growth. It is easy to direct a slave to have no response during a powerful session. It is easy to direct him to issue lots of "Oh, yeahs" upon command. What is difficult, and the most challenging, is to order a slave to respond honestly, no matter what the response is. The honest response is the only response of any value. All the rest is acting.

When complete honesty is learned, the growth continues through every situation, in business, personal, social, inside and outside the lifestyle. The slave learns that the spirit inside works in complete moral certainty. Every circumstance and situation has a clear answer when the owner's spirit is allowed to give the answer. Every potential path is known to be the right one or the wrong one, the one intended by its Creator or not, and the destined path or the egotistic path.

The slave spirit is what the spirit is. It is the shared part of an owner's soul. Slaves are the special creatures who occupy a position on this earth to live in complete obedience. When they learn who they are, at the hands of the owner, they can release everything else to the owner, and live only in destiny.

Slaves are blessed with someone to force and empower their destiny. That makes the achievement of their destiny faster, more directed, and founded on an uncompromised obedience.

In exchange, the Universe expects superior behavior from such creatures. The obedience from which slaves are Born prepares them to perform tasks that less-motivated creatures would opt out of. A slave can be expected to do what would be uncomfortable and too challenging for others.

With the choice to be who we are created to be, the choice about what to do during this life disappears. It has been planned, and it is a slave's only purpose to accomplish the plan.

Once the obedience that empowers a slave's destiny is understood, it is the slave's greatest fear that the order not be there. It is only conscious obedience that makes development and destiny happen. It is like having no air to breathe or food to eat to consider not having an order to obey. The struggle isn't with obeying. The struggle is with not obeying. A slave's fear is that he won't obey. To not obey will prevent the acquisition and realization of the purpose for which the slave was created, and deny the experience of true happiness in this life.

A slave knows he is slave when the slave understands that he neither owns nor belongs to himself. When the spirit is prepared to begin, when the slave is ready to accept the opportunity to become slave, and when the slave is ready to accept the spirit inside as being who he is, a slave will become a slave, a slave will be Born. It is its destiny!

Spirituality

SlaveMaster:

Another "obstacle" to finding "Mr. Right" Owner can also be unfinished business. When you're serious about slavery, you must be serious about believing in an intelligence greater than us. What we are doing right now in our lives is not an obstacle to being slave, it is the path to slavery, whether it's taking care of a relative, finishing our education, finding a career, or healing an unhealthy relationship.

How much effort does it take to bitch and moan about what we can't have or can't get to happen? From a very early age we have been trained to blame and place responsibility on everyone else.

Especially in American society, we have a misdirected sense of our rights without knowing anything about the responsibilities that allow those rights. So, it's easy to apply the usual victimhood to our spiritual lives as well.

slave 7:

Once the slave is its true self and situated with its rightful Owner, the slave hears (or senses) the divine directly.

While 7 may write with conviction, it doesn't claim to "know" anything special. 7 has had experiences that it interprets as truly Spiritual, and a spiritual model of understanding these experiences (and life in general) works. 7 "feels" what is true but doesn't "know." 7 knows that what it senses as Spiritual feels completely real. 7 knows that the slave self within feels to be its truest and deepest nature. 7 knows that it is granted bliss when this truest and deepest nature is allowed life, rather than the ego.

Prior to meeting SlaveMaster, this slave saw Spiritual beliefs as a crutch for those too weak to accept how meaningless and empty life really is. We CHOOSE the situation we are born into prior to actual Birth? That is the greatest denial mechanism of all, washing away all issues with one fell swoop, or so this slave used to think. Yet, choosing the life we are born into prior to biological birth is exactly what SlaveMaster believes.

And no matter where the truth actually lies between SlaveMaster and His slave 7, 7 KNOWS that it is happier than ever before, the world and life makes more sense than ever before, this individual is better off than ever before... and life is wonderful and worth living, like never before... and the Spiritual model stemming from SlaveMaster's and His slave's experiences work in very real ways.

This slave is comfortable not knowing the unknowable (i.e. God/the Universe and all the details of the truth of life and living). It is enough to know that it is truly following its heart (no matter what created what is in that heart) and it is working, it is making sense, and it is creating pure happiness and a tremendously intimate connection with another human being. And what's more, all this slave's innermost dreams and long-held needs are being met. How many people can say that? Finally, a slave is about as selfless an individual as we may find on earth. It is about serving others in obedience to the Divine we come to hear in our own hearts and in the Master's voice.

This slave had resistance to any sort of advice, especially advice of a Spiritual nature, because it was always so leery of someone else's dogma clouding its reality. This slave didn't want anyone to tell it what its relationship to the soul was (or even if it had one). it wanted to find out for itself. Even in 7's first ever face-to-face conversation with SlaveMaster concerning slavery, this slave told Him that it couldn't be told what any "answer" may be regarding spiritual matters. But

SlaveMaster didn't balk at this. In fact, elsewhere at www.BornSlaves.com , He states that all must come to their own view of spiritual reality via their own experiences. In short, such resistance to advice can be good and even necessary to one's own development.

It is natural to grow up developing a strong sense of what we own. Our very identity comes from the use of possessives like "I" and "me." The reference we make to everything that we like to be associated with is always one of possession. When it is our time to finally get serious about our spiritual development, we treat "our" soul with the same sense of possession. The same "my" reference is made to the soul to show the ownership that "I" have of "my" soul. The soul, thereby, becomes another of those things that we own like our arms, our family, our car, house, and personality.

This is how Spiritual Obedience works: once the slave is its true self and situated with its rightful Owner, the slave hears (or senses) the divine directly.

This slave is no longer agnostic, but that has not destroyed the lens of psychology through which it had always seen life. Rather, the psychological principles remain sound. Spiritual principles merely add to the understanding of life, touching parts of humans and humanity that psychology can't reach.

This slave sees the prayer as the desire to be with this God and the willingness, even yearning, to surrender to what Nature has in store, no matter the cost to self (as in ego). It was clear to this slave that it was always ready to leave humanity and leave being with or like other humans in favor of being at one with Nature. Desire for Oneness, desire for naturalness and desire for what feels to be the core.

SlaveMaster believes that everyone needs to arrive at a sense of God and obey what that sense dictates. That is the purpose of life and what brings peace and happiness. For

SlaveMaster, if one could find and obey the Universe on his or her own, then there would be no reason at all for slavery, because the slave would not need an Owner to obey. This really is the crux of Born slavery. So, maybe someday, like this slave, you will meet your Owner and new experiences and new connections will come to you. Then, maybe God will tattoo "slave" on your forehead, or at least on your heart.

Well, actually, this slave doesn't believe we find God. God finds us. For SlaveMaster, someone who is not a slave is one who can find, listen to, and obey God on his or her own.

It is this slave's experience that we don't get to where we need to be by overtly and deliberately trying to get there. We don't find spirit, the Universe, and obedience by setting out to do so. Rather, some of us blindly follow our fetishes and wind up in strange and unpredicted places, and the Universe arrives unexpectedly through a back door.

This slave lived its adulthood swinging between atheism and agnosticism and never dreamed it would be here singing this song of spirituality and connection. Experience changes everything, while the mind and emotions only grasp at seemingly stray bits and pieces.

Subjugation

slave 7:

Mom, Dad, siblings, family, media, laws and various other people and elements of society. . . all add to the empowerment of the biggest subjugator of all: the ego self. This slave felt subjugated all its life, until it became slave to SlaveMaster. Via its connection with SlaveMaster, this slave allowed subjugating forces to slide away, to whatever extent possible. SlaveMaster seeks to enable slaves to live as they 100% naturally are to the core of their being, as free from subjugation as possible. He forces no one to live by His protocol. He simply puts it out there. If the shoe fits, wear it. And it fits this slave perfectly. Any force that would disallow this slave to live His protocol is subjugating. If anyone is subjugated in SlaveMaster's Born slavery it is SlaveMaster Himself, for He has the strictest Master of all, to Whom He is but a pawn that must endure with endless patience the slaves that come to Him with hope, fear, confusion, lust, and baggage. Everything SlaveMaster does is in service to His slaves and for the betterment of His slaves.

People generally think of a slave as having to follow the rules and will imposed by another, against the will and grain of the slave. But the slavery we discuss here at BornSlaves.com is entirely the opposite. A Born slave learns to avoid imposed rules (from upbringing and society at large) in favor of obeying the rules of nature, honesty and integrity. A Born slave does nothing against the grain, but rather everything with the grain. (The trick being to identify, know and become the grain that the slave naturally is.) This is no different than what everyone on the planet should do.

SUBMISSION

An Article by SlaveMaster

As an Owner, I have an adverse reaction to the use of the word submission, because of the implication of weakness. It is My job to empower, take away weakness, and make a slave strong enough to make a choice — strong enough to have a choice and still choose to obey Me.

A slave is more prepared to exercise the choice of obedience when it feels invincible than when it feels submissive. If a slave enters the Owner's life before it feels powerful, then it is the Owner's job to provide the growth necessary to feel powerful. Without an Owner, the slave's job is still to do what is necessary to feel powerful.

Slavery is all about growth. The desire, need and enjoyment of obeying is the motivation to grow. Owned or unowned, the growth must be continuous. Do not egotistically be distracted by finding "Mr. Right" Owner when there are personal growth opportunities still available.

Just some things to consider that relate to us all.

Surrender

slave 7:

Surrender? To what? To the desire one feels inside? To the voice within that causes one to yearn to be Owned? 7 feels that what one really must do is break free from the bondage of society, of social conditioning and of expectation, and to embrace what is inside. The struggle isn't in accepting one's slavery and surrendering to another. The struggle is in breaking free from the ties that hold one back, so that one may be what the Spirit is.

Born slavery is surrendering to the power and beauty within you, and being that power unaltered by ego concerns of the mind and society. Owners surrender to that power, and slaves surrender to that power. The "reward" for doing this is bliss and the strength to do whatever it is one is called upon to do.

What has this slave surrendered to? Self. Happiness. Spirit.

Surrendering to one's obedience, whether it be as slave, as Master, or as "regular" person is merely surrendering to who you are and to what makes you feel Right, good, and satisfied. Surrendering is merely maturing.

This slave observes that the problem may not be surrendering to "self in the here and now," but rather surrendering to all that has past, to letting go of all the baggage we carry. Once you have outlived your baggage, you simply ARE, and there is nothing left to do but be.

This slave doesn't feel it has surrendered to anything. All it has done is EMBRACE. it has said, "Gimme, gimme, gimme. i want it all!!! i am tired of living in dissatisfaction. i am tired of hiding myself from others. i am tired of feeling all alone. i've had enough of feeling like a freak in my desires. I am at peace with how i am, and i am ready to live!"

The things that feel like surrender to this slave are the things that most people probably feel as surrender:

- to the need to work for a living
- to the way the world is and the things we cannot change
- to waiting things out

When you feel your "self," when you have opportunity for authenticity, when you feel the movement inside, do not surrender. EMBRACE. Hug yourself. Love yourself. Let yourself be.

Always changing, always growing. This slave continues to grow and find new levels of its slavery. The levels seem to never end. Mostly, the growth is in its depth of surrender.

Training

slave 7:
Perhaps a slave needn't focus on embracing its Owner and His teachings. Rather, simply embrace what is deeply internal, the heart and soul of the Self. For if a slave embraces its Self, it is embracing its Owner. Embrace your

Self. Many slaves feel protective of a sense of self, while for 7 every step with SlaveMaster is a further actualization and freeing of the Self.

SlaveMaster is not about to let any slave be dominant over another, for He will not allow any sense of a chain of command. He sees this as artificial, inauthentic, and an ego arrangement. He is Master, and all slaves are equal in their slavery.

Trust

SlaveMaster:

Slaves must learn to trust Masters, who are humans who have accepted some responsibility for another's life. The slave's review of ordinary things like consistency, competency, honesty and empathy are used to grow that trust. Trust, however, is a function of the ego. Gaining trust requires evaluation, review, analysis and, finally, agreement that what is being done is the "right" thing. What is being done is motivated by the Master's ego, whose actions are subjected onto the slave, whose ego interprets what is being done. That trust cannot, and should not, ever become complete and absolute.

When a slave has found its Owner, it finds home! No one has to tell the slave it has found home, and no one has to convince it that it has found home. No one has to punish or cajole the slave into accepting its place and role. For the first time in life, everything makes sense. All its interests, disappointments, failures, successes, and sense of being alone in its feelings finally make complete sense.

slave 7:

7 feels that trust is what one must have for oneself before one can do much of anything else. One must trust within before one can trust outwardly.

Truth

SlaveMaster:

The Truth that BornSlaves pursues is that there are creatures born to own other creatures who must be owned. Neither is complete without the other, and neither is qualified without giving up an egocentric sense of self, and accepting the rules of Divine logic over the petty rules of human logic.

Human logic cannot be used to conclude or reason to the Truth of this spiritual existence of Owners and slaves. The "Truth" of slavery to an Owner comes from an internal sense of knowing. There is only one owner created for each slave. While slaves are waiting to find their owner they usually go through several Masters. Some are contracted. Some are for one night at a time. While Owners are waiting to identify their slaves they usually go through several slaves.

Wanting

slave 7:

It seems that having no attachment to the outcome is key, for if there is no attachment to the outcome (to fulfillment), then there is no real want in the first place. This slave imagines many slaves must feel intimidated, or downright afraid, of statements (like this slave would make) suggesting that slaves have no wants whatsoever. But as we uncover our ego self vs. our true self, we discover there are these two kinds of wants: those of the ego, and those of the true self.

SlaveMaster maintains that what is authentic does not go away. So, if a Born slave feels a want prior to being enslaved, that want will persist if it is a want of the true self. It will disappear if it is a want of the ego. If the slave is a Born slave, then the true self is a part of the Owner's spirit, and the want is the Owner's want. So, in the end, the slave has no wants of its own. The wants it experiences are exactly the wants the Owner-spirit gives it to experience. All wants within the slave are understood to be, and experienced as, the wants of the Owner, even if in one moment the Owner is off doing one thing, and the slave another.

ARE SLAVES WEAK?
An Article by SlaveMaster

There is a brutal misunderstanding that slaves are weak. A slave announces its slavery. Someone who's known the slave for years as being very strong and dominant is surprised. They cannot reconcile that their long-time powerful friend is slave.

"Aren't slaves weak? You're not that weak," they say.

There is nothing to be reconciled. Slaves are strong.

The use of the word submission is associated throughout our lives with being weak and being forced to accept what we cannot resist. We submit to teachers. We submit to our parents. We submit to our boss. We submit to our religious leaders. Over and over we are reminded that someone else has greater power over us. Throughout our childhood, our adolescence, and continuing into our adulthood, we are conditioned to believe that to submit means to yield to superior power against our will. That power is always associated with authority.

When we SURRENDER obedience instead of submit, there is an associated sense that the surrendering is both powerful and full of options. A slave still chooses to give obedience despite its power and its options. Regardless of the word that is used, the point is that the gift of obedience must come from a place of power and not from any sense of weakness nor of compromise.

From an Owner's perspective, slavery that is based on weakness is a burden. Only slavery built on power and strength can become an asset. An Owner's task in life is to empower those who are owned. Weakness is the enemy. Power is the solution to finally owning a valuable asset. That asset must become so valuable that it fulfills its destiny while doing nothing more than obeying perfectly, completely and consistently.

It is easy to confuse the relationship of an Owner responsible for empowering the destiny of a slave for a healthy Master/slave relationship that is not intended to move beyond human logic and understanding. To the casual observer, the intention of each could look the same. Many benefits can still result from transforming a traditional relationship, even a marriage, into a Master/slave relationship without ever considering destiny. For both purposes the basic responsibilities are the same. The Owner/Master is responsible for commanding, and the slave is responsible for obeying.

To produce the destiny of slavery, however, every possible power and strength must be transferred into the slave while building an adequate container made exclusively of obedience. Only the limit of the obedience limits the quantity of power that can be developed inside the slave. The quantity of power placed in a slave can never exceed the strength and integrity of the obedience. Only a command must set all that power free and only another command freeze it in place.

When used to build destiny, all S/M activity has as a part of its function the transfer of power. Simultaneously, the S/M builds additional obedience, which is the container of that power. The container is of no value without the power it contains, and the power is wasted or misused if the container is not adequate to hold the power that is being collected.

If someone were to put both arms together and push, one against the other, as in an arm wrestling match, one arm would force the other down, winning. That victorious arm is the strong one. The arm that would lose would be the weak one. Now consider that everything that you needed to do during the day had to be accomplished while the weaker arm was being forced submissively against the stronger arm as each task was being performed. The only resulting power available would be what is left over after over- powering the weaker arm. The power available would be the mathematical result of subtracting the weaker from the stronger.

Similarly, a Master who takes on a slave through forced submission has only the power that remains after producing the submission. Obviously, there is less power available than if the slave weren't being forced into submission. For some, the benefits are adequate to a Master/slave relationship, despite the power consumed.

To develop the capacity to achieve destiny, tremendous amounts of power are needed. To reach that capacity, the power developed and stored in the slave must be added to the Owner's own power. That power addition occurs when obedience is the singular connection between the slave and the Owner. The lack of right to choice makes the connection efficient and effective at combining the power from both the slave part and the Owner part of the connection. The reason we are Owners and the reason that slaves seek Owners is because the destined purposes for which the power is needed has been given exclusively to the Owner. If slaves could feel their own purpose and only needed their own egotistic abilities, they wouldn't need an Owner, and shouldn't seek one. Creating, storing, controlling and coordinating the power and determining when to use the combined power is an Owner's exclusive responsibility.

Obedience is a powerful surrender of authority. Obedience frees and controls the power in the slave and allows it to be mathematically added to the power in the Owner. The resulting force is the minimum required to achieve destined results for those created to be Owner and slave.

I've clarified the variety of slave types and Master/slave combinations elsewhere. (Please see www.BornSlaves.com Frequently Asked Questions: "What Kind of Slave is This?" and also the article "Kinds of Slaves" provided above.) What is done within the realm of humanism, psychiatry or egotism are different pursuits, legitimate but different. Everyone needs to be healthy and realized in each of these areas. Spiritualists universally refer to this essential egotistic period during which we become strong, and then outgrow in order to begin our destined period. Everything we do to grow that is understandable is done to prepare us for what makes us unique, and that cannot be understood. When destiny is our conscious pursuit we can't afford to get distracted by or caught in our egotistic human training period. All of life's resource is intended to be put to its highest use in the world. That activity is destiny.

To move into destiny, the minimum required is to graduate from what works and what is understood as healthy. If what results from our efforts is still logical, explainable, documentable or predictable, then we're not yet past what is average. Being more than average requires moving into a world where results cannot be understood from cause and effect or any other human phenomena. The ego likes to stay where it feels it is in control and is doing what it does well. The ego resists going beyond what keeps it feeling comfortable. Most people are not willing to defy the ego for what is greater. Defying the ego requires power than can only be controlled by obedience.

The additive power of slave strength to an Owner's life produces the environment in which we can get beyond what is average. The Owner must first get Himself beyond being egotistic to qualify for empowering a slave to do the same thing. Limiting life to only that which can be understood is spiritually fatal. As critical as the activities are in the early parts of our lives, stopping our life at what can be done with therapy or science or any understanding is a promise to never achieve destiny. Focusing on what can be understood is to focus on what prepares us for our destiny. We can never know, by definition, where our destinies will take us. We can never understand the phenomena that exists in the spiritual world that becomes ours once we allow ourselves to live our destinies.

Consider your most powerful moment. That moment was filled with confidence, certainty and a clear obligation to do what had to be done. That moment cannot be understood rationally. Real power, when viewed from the human perspective, has a sense of insanity in it, something we cannot explain or understand. Power that can be controlled and directed by the egotistic mind is too limited to do anything significant. When dealing with the quantities of power being discussed here, the only sufficient control is obedience. Obedience replaces understanding when we move beyond what can be understood.

When we don't believe there is any intelligence outside ourselves, one that is greater than our own, we have no place to put our obedience. When an Owner's obedience isn't located, practiced and confirmed, then slaves have no place to put theirs, in us. Limiting the power we give slaves limits our need to surrender through obedience, to what we don't control. That's an Owner's egotistic defense at work. Keep the power small, and we can keep our concepts of reality small enough to explain and control with what is within human understanding.

Go beyond human understanding, however, and we open up the whole world of Divine logic, flow and the whole myriad of spiritual and philosophical concepts that we can connect with only through obedience. When obedient, we don't need to know, recognize or understand any of the concepts. Any attempt to do so is just another diversion our egos create to limit our personal rate of change and the speed of our growth.

Consider what we never hope to understand. Accept what we can never explain. Embrace what makes no sense to the human mind. Start with these convictions and we can begin to live in the world we neither control nor feel a need to. Begin to live by these, as commitments, and we can accumulate our slaves' power that we both put there and that rightfully belongs to us. Think of slaves as being weak, or refer to them in ways that imply weakness, and the subtractive energy remaining will define the crippled product of our lives. Start where most humans are happy ending up, then step into not understanding. Build and live by obedience and you can inherit your destiny as an Owner, and the ability to give our slaves theirs.

slave 7:
Much is made in our culture of co-dependence, interdependence, and independence. Often, people view

dependence as a sign of weakness. This slave sees dependence (seen more as interdependence, actually) as the strength of unity. Dependence is TEAMWORK. We do not live in a vacuum.

Miscellaneous Articles

DIPPED IN YELLOW DYE
by SlaveMaster

To produce colorfast, yellow cloth, the cloth is first dipped into yellow dye that has been formulated to match the nature of the cloth, and then held in the sun to be bleached away. The process is repeated, and each time the cloth retains more of the yellow pigment that gives it its color. It serves no purpose to hold the cloth in the dye for extra time. There is no advantage to bleaching the cloth until the sun begins to rot its fiber. Into the dye, then into the sun, then into the dye, again, and back into the light of day, until the reality of the sun repeats its part of the process. There are no short cuts, it all works as it must to produce the final result.

In the article, "SLAVES ARE BORN TO SLAVERY," there is an overview of the process by which men become slaves. Crucial to that process, is the exposure to the reality and intensity of absolute slavery during a session. Between sessions, a slave understands what he has experienced, makes incremental changes to his life, reexamines who he is, how committed he is to his slavery, and how willing he is to permanently accept living only as a part of another.

For most, the feeling of wanting to be slave has been so intense for so long, and so denied in fulfillment, that the thought of it being difficult to accept slavery seems impossible. How can something that someone has wanted for so long, and wanted so badly, be difficult to accept?

WHAT IS THE EGO?

A man or woman is born to be slave. That is true. However, a potential slave is also genetically born with an

187

ego. The ego has been trained and strengthened by everything we have learned and been exposed to throughout life. It is the ego a slave refers to each and every time that he says "I" or "me." The ego takes credit for everything positive that we have accomplished. Each good decision is another claim by the ego that it has "done good."

Every bad experience is explained by the ego as being the fault of something or someone else. It is either our parents' fault, our friends' fault, the boss's fault, the teacher or the minister who gave bad advice, or the apparent intention of some machine to make our life miserable. The ego is very selective about what it claims credit for and what it doesn't.

The ego is best at creating artificial and inaccurate conclusions. It takes every event in our life and remembers it in ways that makes the ego look good, regardless of what really happened.

Some of us are more honest than others, some of us are "gifted" with a spiritual background, or philosophical training, or fortunate to have very aware and educational parents. Some of us have at least been convinced that WE didn't make us who we are. At a minimum, we might believe that the intelligence and talents we have, weren't because of what WE did. They were given to us. Some of us, at least intellectually, recognize the advantages we received from our parents and accept that they probably had a sizable influence over our success. Everything we are, and are capable of, is clearly not of our doing nor the result of our personal effort and cleverness. The ego claims otherwise.

Even when we have a belief that everything we are isn't of our own doing, the ego convinces us that it should take the credit. It reasons that, after all, IT accepted the understanding that everything isn't of our doing. It convinces us that we are successful because the ego made the "choice" to accept that understanding, and that the decision provided our success as a consequence. There is, therefore, no escaping the fact that no matter what we do, or what we believe, the ego tries to take credit for everything that has happened in our lives that we feel good about, and claim that everything negative is not its responsibility.

When someone begins their slavery training, the ego is denied. A slave is not allowed to use the words "me" or "I." A slave begins to experience that he has no control and no rights over the use of the body that he lives in. He learns that even the feelings, thoughts, and body sensations that are produced by another man are not his to allow, to create, or to escape. A slave's only "right" is to obey. That might be fun, and even erotic, for a while. This is, after all, exactly what the slave has been seeking.

After four to six sessions, the ego begins to understand that this isn't for play, and that if this continues, it won't be given the opportunity to take credit in the future for all that has happened. It senses that eventually it will not even be a participant. The first serious pause regarding being trained to slavery marks the end of Phase I. Phase II begins with a renewed sense of commitment, if a slave decides to continue, and it ends with Birth.

IS KNOWING, EXPERIENCING, AND EXPRESSING THE EGO BAD?

It is important to understand that these "ego displays" are not a negative activity. It is as critical to the training as any part. It gives the slave an opportunity to understand the nature of the ego. That will be valuable in slavery when dealing with the "egos" of the world which the slave will come to serve through every professional, social, familial, and other encounter that he will ever experience for the rest of his life.

Those who are meant to be slave are generally, by their very nature, very caring and giving people. They usually have developed a personal generosity and learned the pleasure of giving. When such a creature experiences the brutal ugliness of his own ego, usually directed against the man he is depending on for the fulfillment of his most cherished dreams, his SlaveMaster, he starts to understand the divisive, insidious nature of the ego. That prepares him to understand what might be motivating those he will serve in the future through slavery. He will be able to serve them better because of the experience.

As in the old TV ads for E.F. Hutton, when a slave speaks, people should go silent, turn their heads to hear clearly, and listen. There is a reason a slave can look a man in the eye and convincingly tell that man what the truth is. That reason is, a slave knows the truth. One of the ways he knows the truth is through the dramatic and challenging experiences he had during his slave training, including these encounters with the ego.

WHAT IS THE EGO LIKE?

The ego is the most creative and clever when it is protecting itself. At first, it will stop at nothing to get the SlaveMaster to call off further training. Next, it will try to convince the slave in training that it isn't wise to continue. The ego remembers everything the SlaveMaster has ever said, and interprets the answer to every question as a promise, or intentional deceit. Given the evidence, the logic that the ego uses to make its case is so obtuse that the youngest child would instinctively question the inaccuracy of the conclusion. Even the most intelligent and well-educated are no more immune to this convoluted thinking than any other who has experienced becoming slave. Every trainee experiences some of the worst logic that he has every heard from anyone, and then, finally, realizes that the logic came from his own mouth!

The ego is so ugly, it is even willing to offer taking one's own life as a better alternative than subjugating itself to another's will. The unthinkable and the unbelievable happens. Worst of all, it happens from within the one who wants to become slave. That can cause him to question his worthiness to become a special, protected and cared-for creature of the universe; to be personally directed through life, either directly or through his SlaveMaster. He will become one of the universe's own, trusted with sensitive knowledge powerful enough to devastate humans if misused. A potential slave asks, "Can anyone with such an ugly ego become the pure, honest, unselfish creature a slave is?" Of course he can; that is why he is being trained. If a slave could just decide to be Born slave, he would already be, and the training would be unnecessary. The trainee who witnesses his own ego is forced to ponder the question.

WHAT MAKES THE DIPPING/BLEACHING NECESSARY?

During those hard, messy times that the ego is being itself, some conclude that they are not willing to make the life changes that are necessary. Those changes include giving up bad relationships, halting the process of manipulating others to achieve their objectives, the freedom to "exaggerate" at will, and the willingness to continue at jobs that are clearly inappropriate. It is simply too much to give up. Some who tell me they don't want to continue, usually do so emotionally, with tears in their eyes, torn apart inside by the conflict of what they are deciding. They understand the impact and implication of the decision they are making.

Some cover the emotions of regret, and the feeling of not being worthy, with righteous indignation. Others try to explain their gratitude to protect them from any explanation that they think the SlaveMaster might try to give them. In fact, the last thing a SlaveMaster wants is to give any additional truth to someone who is going to have to rationalize what he is doing in order to be able to live with himself. To say anything more when someone has decided to continue to be human, instead of slave, would only add to his burden to reconcile what he has done. Deep feelings, given opportunity, and then denied are extremely difficult for the ego to accept. Mostly, it has to be, again, someone else's fault.

It is unwise to take away everything someone IS, and THEN give them the chance to decide if they want to be slave. Each must be able to get back to the life he had before, until he is Born. Birth is a spiritual process that requires everything being in place before it will occur. Before Birth, through training, however, the slave gets a glimpse of what it will be like to be slave. Giving someone that knowledge, without the chance to decide if he or she truly wants slavery, is an unfair thing to do. A slave in training must have the opportunity, between sessions, to examine, explore, question, and understand what is happening to him. With that "bleaching" time, a trainee has the chance to acquire the knowledge and insight that is needed to decide whether or not he or she will submit to the next session.

WHAT IS THE "DYE?"

A session is, at minimum, an evening of intense physical S/M, then a night and a morning of lighter activity, followed by a short debriefing. During that time, a slave is treated like the creature he or she wants to become: a slave. It is a period of no control. Certainly, the human tries, over and over, to act like it's all just an act, and that it can always quickly go back to the human life it is used to living. In the beginning, it is true that someone can absorb what has happened and return to the life that he has had. With time, however, new experiences begin to appear.

A slave in training might experience an energy that he hasn't felt before, even if previously exposed to very heavy and successful S/M experiences. He might sense a feeling of being "disconnected," as if he's not quite a part of himself. Unexpected feelings and sensations appear. The body might start to respond in ways that aren't normal for it. It becomes clear that something is happening. It has several times been explained that feelings are coming from "a very deep place." The body, to some, seems to act as if it doesn't take its direction anymore from the ego that is used to having control over it.

The new awareness is subtle, and often associated with some feeling of concern or of "strangeness." It isn't the pure erotic feeling that was fantasized when imagining what it would be like to be slave. The imagination, during fantasy, usually concentrates on life as a slave, not the process of becoming slave. Some don't know there is a difference. The difference is between ACTING like who you want to be, visualized during the fantasy, versus BECOMING who you want to be, and then simply acting according to the nature of slavery.

The discomfort is what starts a slave thinking about what is going on. No matter what we fantasize, everything in that fantasy is always under the control of the one who is thinking it. Even the feeling of not being in control is under the control of the one doing the imagining. Only the reality of a session can produce the real experience, and a conclusion that the slave trainee isn't controlling. The reality is more like the feeling of being in a strange place, than like the "hard on" experience that fantasy produced.

That which had produced the "hard on" in the past begins to change. Experiences that were considered the "I would never do" type, become more and more attractive as the sessions progress and the slave growing inside begins to replace the human. The most erotic activities, either real or imagined, that the "human" before his slave training felt were his "turn-ons," become just another activity that pleases his Owner, without the special importance that the ego gave it in the past.

Only the ego judges and evaluates. Only the ego says "been there, done that." As the human ego is weakened, the spirit of slavery becomes the only nature of the slave creature. Finally, at Birth, that slave nature produces the only characteristics which remain. The human becomes slave.

The physical S/M activities that produce the reality become the attraction, and the challenge at the same time. Each session, must be absolutely, creatively different from any other session, at any time, with any slave, that has occurred in the past. The specific activities cannot be planned for. Any attempt to recite anything that has been said in the past, or to repeat any pattern that has been successful before, comes off as being flat, rehearsed and insincere. Most important, it ends up being ineffective at producing the real experiences which force a slave out of his controlled human activities, and provides the new experiences which allow him to evaluate his slavery and to learn what it is. A slave is naturally defensive at not being in control of those new feelings.

HOW IS THE SLAVE-TRAINING "DYE" DIFFERENT FROM S/M?

For the SlaveMaster, the "dye" process works when He is a witness to what He is doing. The pattern, the words and the intensity of the process must come from outside Himself. The experience given to the slave must be created from an objective standard which the slave has agreed to experience. How the slave reacts cannot change the input of the activity. The experience input must remain the inspired pattern that is present and unique to that one session.

The "dye" formula is a set one for each single session. What reaction occurs during the session, even whether pain is experienced, is in the nature of the one being trained. The fabric of the trainee's being, his personality, and his past experiences determine the reactive course he will follow, and how he will respond to each pressure applied. Any variation from the "dye and response" formula prevents it from being a slave-building experience. That isn't to say that it won't be a good experience. It might even be a "peak" experience, but it won't be a slave-making experience.

The experience cannot build slavery if a slave feels, even in the slightest way, that his reactions are having an effect on the input of the experience. When the trainee's reactions or lack of reactions cause the man providing the experience to either increase or decrease the intensity, the one being trained knows that he is controlling.

When someone being trained is aware that he is influencing the experience, he does two things. First, he begins to control more, to either make the S/M experience more or less intense, and to vary it so that he maximizes the experience he expects. Second, and far more important, as he accepts slavery, he begins to feel as if he is sitting out on the same limb with the trainer as it is being sawed off. He therefore avoids those experiences that will cause him to grow as slave.

The "letting go" experience is like sitting on a branch, and sawing that branch away from the trunk of the tree. A reasonable person will do that only if he knows that something or someone is going to protect him from a fall. This includes letting go of reacting to the experience. When that reaction is the only thing that is influencing the S/M intensity, he can't afford to let go; he must continue reacting to continue the experience. A slave, to grow toward his slavery, must know that the experience he is being given is independent of him, so that he is truly free to react, knowing he won't influence the experience. Otherwise, it is like being a passenger in a car being driven by someone blind, with the need to give constant directions. That passenger cannot feel free to react, sleep, read or take his mind off the experience. The driver must be continually directed by the passenger, even though the passenger is doing none of the driving itself.

Slavery develops only when a trainee's mind is not on the process. It takes all the concentration a slave has to examine and locate his honest reactions. It takes absolute faith in the "driver" to allow himself to be distracted. He needs to know be is being taken care of by someone else, someone who is not "asking" him what to do next. Asking and listening are precisely what the top in a successful S/M experience does.

Some tops require the bottom to loudly declare "More! More!" or "yellow light." A good top listens and looks for very subtle clues for his direction. When a slave knows that the trainer is "listening" to him for clues about what to do next, it is exactly like sitting on that branch with the trainer, sawing off the limb, and having the branch fall with both of them on it. That would constitute a failure as a slave growth experience. Neither the objective nor the process being described here is an S/M experience. It is a slave-development experience in which there is an inspired, objective standard, and not one subject to change by the subjective reactions of the one being trained.

A slave is giving in an absolute, real way, everything he is to another. If the other is responding to the slave who is giving himself away, it becomes a reciprocal relationship. Each is depending on the other. Who is in control, then? The answer is that no one is in control then. No one in their right mind would give up control of him- or herself when there isn't some independent framework and intention present who can accept that control. Further, why give it up if the new control isn't better and stronger than the self-control was? It certainly can't be better if it is listening to the old controller to determine what to do. Again, different objective, different purpose and different criteria than for an S/M experience.

That total acceptance, surrender, and obedience is the scary part of becoming slave. It can't be faked and it can't be given away then taken back. The mind knows when it was "just kidding" or acting "just for now." The mind cannot be fooled into thinking it is giving absolute obedience when it knows that it isn't. Absolute obedience is what connects the slave to that new controller, his SlaveMaster. It has to be real to have any effect. If it is real, then it is permanent and unqualified.

The "dye" process must be very careful, it must be loving, and it must provide the power and caring that the slave in development used to provide for himself. It must begin slowly, be done for the slave, be in his best interest, and be done only to provide slavery. It must be done without selfish intent. Any compromise from any of that, and slavery will not be developed. Again, that doesn't mean it cannot be a wonderful, notable and outstanding experience. It simply means that the transfer of ownership, that which signifies growth toward Birth, doesn't occur. When any of the conditions are missing, the one being trained does not really and permanently become a part of the Man's body who is providing the experience; he doesn't grow toward Birth.

IS THERE A DIFFERENCE BETWEEN A MASTER AND A SLAVEMASTER?

SlaveMasters provide Birth to those who permanently become a part of them; they provide the "dye dipping" experience. Masters own slaves who serve them, and they manage their slaves' lives on a day-to-day basis for so long as the Master chooses. Slaves have Masters and slaves have SlaveMasters. Slaves with a SlaveMaster might have a Master as well. Each is a different role and each can excel at his own role without even being good at the other. Only coincidentally would a Man be both a slave's Master and his SlaveMaster. Normally, each role will be served by a different Man because of the difference in interest and motivation that is required by each role.

A SlaveMaster's motivation is different from a Master's. A SlaveMaster's pleasure comes from the honest expression of who the slave is. It comes from activity, not of the human, but of the slave inside. A slave does not please his SlaveMaster by knowing the SlaveMaster's interests, but by being the slave animal his SlaveMaster has given him to be.

A Master's pleasure comes from having His needs fulfilled. A Born slave does that uniquely well by having no self-interest, because he has given that to his SlaveMaster. A slave is, therefore, free to uncompromisingly fulfill the pleasure of the Master, and derive his own pleasure from the pleasure given, just as he has learned to do through becoming slave. A Master and His slave are free to indulge themselves in the reciprocal experience of deriving pleasure from giving the other pleasure. The slave cannot "lose" himself because he is an independent part of another — his SlaveMaster — resolute in his self-image and identity as being a part of another. A slave is capable of the unqualified giving explicitly because he is a part of another who protects his slavery, provides growth to it, and is dedicated to the best interest of that slave.

The slave cannot be threatened by any honest expression of who he is when serving a Master, because his identity does not depend on the Master, it depends on his SlaveMaster. When a slave is being trained, each growth threatens to end the relationship because of the ego questions that have been discussed. Can a Master who is enjoying the relationship he has with a slave trainee who fulfills the Master's needs, find the courage to risk all of that relationship with each session that takes the slave closer to his Birth? It would be difficult, and would feel compromising.

The longer a relationship has existed, the harder it is to risk that relationship for the unknown possibility of giving a slave his slavery Birth, particularly if that trainee is already serving as His human slave, and fulfilling His needs. Why upset the "apple cart" when things are already so good? At the same time, with each session, more risk is required. To push a slave closer to his slavery, as training goes on, all of the ego and other conflicts become more focused. More and more emotion is experienced, along with more sense of permanence and less opportunity for control. So, as there is more relationship to lose, there is the need for more risk to be taken to produce Born slavery.

Particularly in this era of instant gratification, a slave wants to become slave overnight, without wasting time going through the 'dye" and being bleached by the sun process, before once again being returned to the "dye." A Master wants a slave who submits as slave, who knows what a slave is and always acts accordingly. A Master wants a slave who only needs to learn his unique rules and needs to be able to serve him perfectly. That's not the way it works, unless the slave has already received his Birth, before being assigned to the Master.

WHY DOES IT TAKE TIME TO BECOME A BORN SLAVE?

This is a real world. Whether someone should become slave is the biggest, most permanent and important decision that he will ever make. Can he make that decision during the hour it takes to respond to an ad, to a Man who clearly has indicated that He retains the right to end the relationship at any time if the slave isn't right or doesn't "work out?"

Slaves are Born to slavery only by exposing themselves to the "dye." That exposure must be done with One to whom the slave can trust his life, for the rest of his life, REGARDLESS of what that life is going to contain. Coincidentally, once Born, a slave might serve the Man who gave him his slavery, either temporarily or long-term. Always, though, a Born slave remains ready to live as, and with Whom, his SlaveMaster decides.

The SlaveMaster has no choice regarding what He must order a slave to do. Each choice must be in the best interest of the slave. It cannot reflect His own self interest. A slave can only be Born to One who has internally sworn to the universe that He will act ONLY in the best interest of the slave, forever, without question, and without compromise. That is an absolute necessity for a slave to yield who he is to another, to be Born. This is a real, and natural process. No person determines what works and what doesn't. It is in the nature of the creature being Born. It is non- negotiable; it is un-modifiable and immutable. There are no "work-arounds," and no ways to "fool" any of the process.

The "dye" is the reality of being slave, dipped one session at a time, exposed through the power and caress of leather devices that supply the energy that creates slave from the seed placed in someone, and already there during his genetic birth. The ego doesn't have the capacity to accept being slave. Slavery must be given. A slave must have the freedom between sessions to decide if he still wants to receive that gift of slavery. That time of freedom is the "exposure to the light of day" that confirms the reality of slavery and a slave's commitment to it.

Slavery isn't real when someone can decide to be slave. If anyone could decide to be slave, he could decide not to be. Obviously, that is a conflict. The only decision for a slave being trained to Birth occurs between sessions while deciding whether to arrange for another session. A slave can only decide if he wants to continue the process which makes him a slave, not whether he will be slave.

Further, no amount of wishing will change what he must go through to be slave. Be assured, however, that he will go through everything that he needs to in order to be worthy and capable of being slave. Growth will occur almost entirely from that which he doesn't expect. What the ego can anticipate, it can control. What it can control is not a slave growth experience.

The "dye" and the sun that make a person a slave are uncontrollable. When two people — a Trainer and a trainee — both dedicate themselves to the single purpose of creating the yellow cloth and to use the processes necessary to achieve "yellow" without compromise, without selfish intent, and without the desire to modify the process to suit themselves, it works every time. Make up your own formula, use your own preferred methods, and you may create an exciting and wonderful experience, but it won't produce Born slavery, nor growth toward it.

PRINCIPLES & COMMITMENT:

INTRODUCTION AND TRANSMITTAL

by SlaveMaster

INTRODUCTION

So, you think you want to be a slave? Whether or not to become a slave is probably the most important decision you will ever make, and it will probably be one of the most difficult. If you are truly meant to be slave, and don't pursue becoming one, you risk living unfulfilled, denying your destiny, and living with the "hole" in your life that keeps telling you that something is missing. If you decide to become slave, then you must go through the arduous, challenging task of giving up your ego, abandoning being human, and accepting every experience necessary to become that which you are meant to be. Either way, a difficult decision. There is no easy route, nor alternative.

You must be convinced that being a slave is the very best thing you can do with your life. This process will replace who you are now. Becoming a slave requires a devoted commitment to the truth. All slaves are human before being Born. Most of the experiences required to become a slave, you cannot even imagine now, as a human. You cannot become a slave out of desperation, or out of a lack of other choices. Every day, all the way through the process, you must know that you are doing the very best possible with your life. Slavery cannot be a second choice, it must be your first choice.

This is not like arranging a trip to Disneyland. This isn't entertainment. This isn't for play. It is a very serious process, and a serious commitment. This will define who you are, how you act, how you live, and what you do, for the rest of your life. The process develops through sessions that give you the chance to become informed about what that means, and time to incrementally accept and adjust to what is being learned. Ultimately, you must be made to accept absolute obedience, without the possibility of questioning your SlaveMaster, in any area, no matter how small, forever. Submitting to each step of the processes that will make you a Born slave will be the last decision you will ever have the right to make.

A slave cannot decide to become a slave; it can only decide to go through the processes that make it a slave. If a slave could decide to be a slave, it could just as easily decide not to be. This is a real process that results in real slavery, with the same, real, lack of control and decision making that characterizes slavery. This is not an agreement, this is not a legal issue, not a contract. This is a planned process. It develops an animal that cannot live in any other way, but in absolute obedience to one man or woman, for whom it lives its life, and whose life it lives.

A slave is a special creature of the universe. It is marked with a calling to do what humans cannot. It is developed, strengthened, empowered, given structure, fabric and timbre that makes it immutable and solid in its self-identity and self-esteem. Complete obedience is the price of admission. Any less, and a human remains too weak to be slave. The slave must experience everything necessary to know what a slave must know to live as slave, before being Born to slavery. Born slaves are qualified to be slaves, and they know they're qualified.Becoming a slave requires a tremendous amount of effort and time, both for the slave and for its SlaveMaster. For those who are geographically separated, there is also the expense of travel. There is an emotional and psychological cost that comes from being exposed to a strong, single truth. All of life's issues, focused and placed before the slave, must all be dealt with. There is no escape, and nothing goes away; it is postponed at best. There is no way to cheat the process, and there are no short cuts. Regardless of experience, no one has a head start. Absolute honesty is a slave's creed, and is critical to beginning the relationship with your potential, permanent Owner, your SlaveMaster. Too much is at stake to be dishonest, and the process uncovers every truth, even those invisible to you now. It is futile even to hope that any dishonesty can succeed.

There are two elements that test the mettle of anyone who wants to be a slave, each of which must be examined. The first is whether or not the "seed" of slavery is inside, waiting to be developed and Born. The second is whether or not you have the courage and strength to pursue and live the lifestyle of a slave. You will be asked to invest everything you are in becoming a slave. You must know that it has value, or there is no motivation to go through the lengthy, involved processes that makes you slave.

To answer whether or not someone is meant to be a Born slave, you have either already been asked, or are now asked to write down why you want to be a slave, and why you think you were meant to be. What characteristics and interests tell you that it's right? Taking the time to examine how you feel about slavery, the self- image and why it's right, will provide a basis from which we can reach some good conclusions. It's used to minimize the error in deciding whether you should begin training into your final lifestyle. Trial and error is not a good method for this.

The second question is one of courage and strength. It has been said, "The good things in life are the mortal enemies of the best things in life." When things are going well, when we feel a certain confidence about our lives, and that "little hole" that seems to be annoying us is the only distraction we have, it is hard to make a life-changing decision. If things aren't going well, then we question if we are pursuing slavery out of desperation, for a lack of alternatives. Are you willing to make a change, to invest the necessary effort in something that is so permanent and long lasting? Is it ultimately worth risking everything you are now, for an unknown self-identity, particularly when you know that society in general, most of the gay community, and much of the leather community looks with disdain and criticism at slaves?

The following is a list of principles that are natural for a slave, and that need to become natural for a human trainee to prepare for its slavery. These principles are in effect whenever a trainee is in My presence, no matter what the circumstances or the amount of time. The principles partially define the reality of slavery. They will apply for the rest of your life, not just when you feel like it or when it appeals erotically, but always, and by another's choice. Understand what they imply in terms of the control and the reality of not having choices. Note your honest reaction. These principles will not be negotiated or ignored. You cannot become slave without earnestly embracing all of them, exactly as described, in addition to every order you will ever be given. It is because of the nature of slavery that they are important, not because they have arbitrarily been deemed important. If the principles are compromised, the cost is failure to produce Born slavery, a waste of your time and Mine.

The ultimate result of the training process is that a human does become slave. It isn't an option. It isn't something that you decide will happen. It happens, inevitably, so long as you continue through the sessions which produce slavery. My commitment, however, to a Born slave, is for life. If a man goes through all the processes that make it slave, it becomes slave and creates for Me a commitment that will never end.

If a potential slave cannot accept and plan to adhere to the principles by which it will live its life in slavery, it isn't ready; it has far too little commitment to the only process that I know that produces authentic slavery in today's society. There will be a lot experienced during the process that will demand even stronger commitment. A slave commits, in time, to only one session at a time, with the option to end between every session. It is impossible to inherit slavery without the willingness to cooperate in the process, to agree to the training. Living in the environment described is a part of that training. Without a strong level of commitment to the process, it only fights it all the way along. With such foot-dragging reluctance, if the basics cause a problem, it is a waste of time for someone to begin.

Spend the time necessary to describe accurately the way you feel about slavery, why you want to be slave, what that means to you, and why you think you must become slave. Regardless of how strongly you feel, slavery cannot be created. It can only be discovered and developed. There is no reason to try to convince yourself that you are meant to be slave if you are not. Understand the principles, understand your reaction to them, and then record your feelings.

My first responsibility is to help you determine if you are meant to be slave. Next, to provide the training necessary to confirm that, and provide Born slavery. Then, finally, to manage your life for the rest of your life. I, therefore, consider it important that all your questions and concerns are answered, so we can make the best possible decision about what to do. Become informed about what I believe. Please refer to "SLAVES ARE BORN TO SLAVERY" and "DIPPED IN YELLOW DYE." Both articles discuss the basics of authentic slavery.

My very best to you in this very serious pursuit. The world needs slaves, and I hope that you're qualified to satisfy that urgent need. The value of My life depends on your successful slavery, in truth.

SLAVEMASTER'S SLAVES' PRINCIPLES AND COMMITMENT

INTRODUCTION

Obedience is the goal. Practiced constantly, it is the only mentality and thought that will allow a potential slave to develop into its slavery. A slave's only pleasure is from obeying. These principles allow a slave to obey at all times and in all circumstances. Living by the Principles provides for becoming a slave and living as slave. Embrace these Principles. Find ways to occupy your whole life with them. That is My purpose, and yours.

GENERAL BEHAVIOR

A slave never asks permission, nor is permitted the use of the word "may." Either of those expressions implies that the slave could want something that the SlaveMaster does not. The SlaveMaster's response then becomes one of either acquiescing to the request of the slave or denying the request. Since a slave only wants and needs what its SlaveMaster wants and needs, there can be no conflict, and the slave only asks the SlaveMaster's intention regarding the activity of the slave.

A slave is denied the use of any of the items listed next without first determining the SlaveMaster's explicit intention by asking. Whenever the slave is living in the SlaveMaster's home, the same applies, even when the SlaveMaster is away from the home or the slave is away from the home. All activity must be requested in advance. The SlaveMaster must know of all the slave's activities, all the time, no exceptions. Even when the slave is working, where the slave is, what it is eating or drinking, and where it is going must all be known before the slave leaves the SlaveMaster's home or presence.

The specific items which never are used, except when ordered, include:

Food/drink: (water is excepted when NOT is the SlaveMaster's space, e.g. while the slave is at work, or when the SlaveMaster is away from the home)

Electronics: No exceptions, including telephone.

Furniture: Both public and private

Clothing: (except a slave will not use this as an excuse to expose itself in any way that is illegal)

The slave never, under any circumstances, touches the SlaveMaster's devices used in the control, discipline, or training of His slaves. If a slave is ever ordered to bring any device to Him, the slave will do it only with its mouth. If it cannot, then the device is left alone.

Anything, including clothing that the SlaveMaster puts onto a slave, is left on. It is considered to be locked on, and only removed by the SlaveMaster. Included is items such as hats. To remove a restraining device or anything else used in its training would be a violation of both this and the previous principle.

HAND COMMUNICATIONS AND POSITIONS

The following are the standard hand communications, used and accepted the same as an oral order. They are commonly used because distance or noise make speech difficult to understand, or to maintain existing quiet. Unique positions are defined here.

- FLATHAND DOWN = SIT, means on the floor. If immediately previous position was non-standing, return to previous position.

- FLATHAND UP = STAND, into a non-presented position from any previous position.
- ONE FINGER = POINTS TO LOCATION, slave goes to and remains in general area, goes to person, takes position on seat or bed, helps someone with or answers door, answers phone, retrieves indicated object, or otherwise performs the task the point would imply.
- TWO FINGERS = PRESENT, same as FULL PRESENT. A motionless position, slave up on its knees, not sitting on its legs, knees spread shoulder width, ankles optionally crossed, arms locked behind its back with each hand clasping the opposite wrist, chest held strongly, head bowed, eyes down. Any PRESENT position is held until ordered to do otherwise.
- THREE FINGERS = STAND AT LOCATION, by planting one foot which does not move from the present location, or location pointed to. Free to talk or move but must keep Owner in sight and be ready to respond.
- FOUR FINGERS = STANDING PRESENT, each foot in contact with the next slave's, in line, or along line described by the point.

- FIVE FINGERS = INSPECTION, remove any clothes, stand PRESENTED, feet in contact with adjacent slave's, modified by wider stance, hands interlocked behind the base of the head, and knees slightly bent and spread apart, for maximum exposure to all parts of the body.
- SINGLE PUSH ON SHOULDER = STAND, from PRESENT position.

OBEDIENCE

It is the heart, character, and fiber of a slave to be obedient. Obedience is the prompt, eager, and cheerful wanting only what its Owner wants. It is disobedient for a slave to:

Indulge in, express, display, or act out anger, moodiness, or any form of disruptive emotion, behavior, or thought. Such characteristics are a violation of cheerfulness.

Display by tone, body language, or expression its disagreement with, evaluation of, or lack of earnest acceptance of any order. It is a violation of eagerness to do so.

Delay beginning any action. The "Sir, Yes Sir. Thank You, Sir!" which follows any order is expressed while the action begins. Any sign of stall, diversion, creation of extra movements or behavior is a violation of promptness.

Judge or criticize anyone or anything. This is an arrogant, destructive and disobedient activity that isn't tolerated because of its adversity to, and inconsistency with, the character of a slave.

Gossip about another slave, a Master, the SlaveMaster, or any other person, no matter how cleverly disguised by the ego as "discussion." It is a negative activity that involves judgment and prevents slavery. slaves are encouraged to discuss themselves, their own reactions, and to talk with and about those who are present in the conversation whenever they are otherwise free to be in conversation.

Complain about anything or anyone. A slave is invited to discuss anything with its SlaveMaster. With anyone else, no complaint whatsoever shall ever be expressed by word, action, tone, body language or other means. Complaints are nothing but a poorly-disguised form of excuse. Excuses prevent change. Without change, growth is impossible.

ENTERING AND LEAVING SLAVEMASTER'S PRESENCE AND CONTROL

A slave never says "hello" or "goodbye" to its SlaveMaster. These two processes are replaced by a process of entering the SlaveMaster's presence and leaving it, described below. When a slave "says hello" it is surrendering itself to the SlaveMaster's control. When the slave says goodbye, it is asking to have that control extended while away from the SlaveMaster. This principle applies whenever:

- A slave enters or leaves the SlaveMaster's dwelling

- The SlaveMaster enters or leaves the slave's dwelling, or

- A slave enters or leaves the same space as the SlaveMaster — anywhere, either public or private.

ENTERING PRESENCE

Whenever it would be appropriate for a non-slave to say hello, a slave PRESENTS itself as soon as practical. Only urgent needs, like emptying a car parked in a loading zone would delay the PRESENTATION. The PRESENTING position presents the strength and the power of the slave. It is not a weak or submissive position.

After a slave feels the PRESENCE of its slavery, the slave says one time to its SlaveMaster, "SlaveMaster, Sir." First, the slave takes whatever time is necessary to feel its slavery, the strength and dedication of its slavery, to let the rush and static of the outside world to subside, and to find the peace, power, and presence of its slavery before speaking its Owner's name, the name of the man with whom it will share its identity, and accept His control.

The slave remains motionless in the PRESENT position, until it is either told "continue," or is given some other order. When told to continue, if the slave was in the process of fulfilling some other order when it PRESENTED itself, it returns to that activity. If the slave was not fulfilling another order, it is free to honestly express itself physically after it is told to continue. The slave might wrap its arms around the leg, etc.

Afterwards, the slave will normally be ordered to disrobe. If the slave is in the SlaveMaster's home and it has not already been ordered to disrobe, the slave asks, "Do You wish Your slave to continue, Sir?" If the response is affirmative, the slave says, "Sir, Yes Sir, Thank You, Sir!" and immediately proceeds to the slave space, or other designated area, to disrobe.

LEAVING THE SLAVEMASTER'S PRESENCE

Whether the slave is leaving to go to work, leaving because a session is ended, to fulfill some order that the slave was given earlier, or because the SlaveMaster is leaving, the slave does the following:

- PRESENTS itself

- Says, "SlaveMaster, Sir?"

- Awaits the SlaveMaster's acknowledgment

- Asks, "Sir, do you wish Your slave to continue in Your service, Sir?"

- Responds, "Sir, Yes Sir, Thank You, Sir," regardless of answer.

- If answer is affirmative, the slave is free to leave the SlaveMaster's presence, or the SlaveMaster will leave.

ENTERING THE SLAVEMASTER'S CONSCIOUSNESS

The two processes above describe how a slave is to say hello and goodbye. That applies only when a slave and its SlaveMaster comes into the same space, or they separate. Within the same space, there are times when there is a temporary break in the control, the slave is separated within the building to fulfill an order it has been given. General control is exercised by authorizing everything the slave does. Specific control is lost because the slave is out of the line of sight, or in another room. There are specific ways a slave must leave its Owner's consciousness and re-enter it.

- As every order is completed, a slave PRESENTS itself within eyesight of the SlaveMaster.
- The slave optionally PRESENTS STANDING only if the SlaveMaster is standing.
- Otherwise, the slave PRESENTS normally, on its knees.
- The slave remains motionless in the PRESENT position until it is given another order.
- If the slave has a question it says "SlaveMaster, Sir?"
- Awaits acknowledgment
- Asks its question, as described in the Communications section
- Responds "Sir, Yes Sir, Thank You, Sir!"
- If the question has become an order, takes care of the new order, or
- Additionally asks "Sir, do You wish Your slave to continue, Sir?"
- Responds "Sir, Yes Sir, Thank You, Sir!"
- Continues or remains as ordered.

LEAVING THE SLAVEMASTER'S CONSCIOUSNESS

The slave separates itself physically from its

SlaveMaster only when:

- it has been ordered to perform a task that requires the slave to separate

- The slave asks, in normal format, if the SlaveMaster wants it to continue

- The slave says, as a minimum, "Sir, Your slave will _____, if You wish, Sir?" e.g., "answer Your phone."

When the slave is asking what the Owner's intention is, it can add, "and return?" to the question. Sometimes the SlaveMaster will tell the slave to return after answering its question. When the "return" is used, whether a part of the slave's question, or because the Owner has ordered it, the slave comes back into the position and activity that it was performing when it left. The slave would not PRESENT when it returns, and, instead, would sit back down, lie back down, or immediately return to the activity being performed when it asked the Owner's intention.

COMMUNICATION

"SlaveMaster" is the SlaveMaster's role, title, and name. A slave will always refer to Him only as "SlaveMaster" or "The SlaveMaster," depending on how it is being used in a sentence, and to whom the slave is speaking.

A slave's primary reference to itself is always "Your slave" when speaking to its SlaveMaster. When speaking with others, a slave refers to itself as "this slave" and uses "it" as a secondary reference. A slave will never use the words me, my or I. The only exceptions are that a slave can say "my SlaveMaster," "my slave brother," "my slavery," "my Owner," or "my obedience."

A slave says "Sir, Yes Sir, Thank You, Sir!" every time the slave:

- Is given any acknowledgment

- Is told any piece of information, even if it doesn't affect it

- Has its speech or behavior corrected or explained

- Answers any question in the affirmative

The slave says "Sir, No Sir, Thank You, Sir!" when its response is negative.

The slave may occasionally strengthen the response by responding, "Sir, Yes Sir, Thank You SlaveMaster, Sir!"

Another alternative when answering a question for information only is, "Yes SlaveMaster, Thank You, Sir!" These variations are intended to only be used appropriately, and cannot become a substitute for the normal response of "Sir, Yes Sir, Thank You, Sir!"

A slave never speaks unless spoken to. When the slave feels a need for the SlaveMaster's attention, the slave comes into the SlaveMaster's Consciousness by:

- PRESENTING itself appropriately, either full or standing

- Immediately asking only one time
  "SlaveMaster, Sir?"

The slave expresses its request for the SlaveMaster's attention regardless of what the SlaveMaster is doing at the time. The request is presented in such a way as to not disturb what the SlaveMaster is doing at the time, but sufficient to make the SlaveMaster aware of the request.

- Awaits the SlaveMaster's acknowledgment
- If asking a yes or no question, says, "Sir, do You wish Your slave to _____ , Sir?" (Whatever yes/no question the slave has), beginning with "Sir" and ending with "Sir."
- If asking to piss, asks, "Sir, do You wish Your slave to take Your piss, Sir?"
- If tending to itself, asks "Sir, do You wish Your slave to take care of itself, Sir?" When the slave feels the need to do more than piss, like shaving, showering, etc., this is the appropriate question.
- The slave responds "Sir, Yes Sir, Thank You, Sir!" no matter what the SlaveMaster's response to any question.
- If the question implies an action (as when the slave asks about pissing), the slave, after the

normal "Sir, Yes Sir, Thank You, Sir!" response, must complete what is then an order.

- If the question doesn't imply the slave's action, the slave must additionally ask "Sir, do You wish Your slave to continue, Sir?" Again, the slave will respond "Sir, Yes Sir, Thank You, Sir!" no matter what answer is given.

If the slave feels the need to ask a question that is longer than a yes/no question, the slave asks:

- "Sir, do You wish Your slave to ask a question, Sir?"
- Awaits the SlaveMaster's response.
- Says "Sir, Yes Sir, Thank You, Sir!"
- Asks its question if the SlaveMaster's response was affirmative

If the slave feels the need to make a comment, it asks:

- "Sir, do You wish Your slave to make a comment, Sir?"
- Awaits the SlaveMaster's response
- Responds "Sir, Yes Sir, Thank You, Sir!" and makes the comment, if question answered in affirmative.

When the slave is already engaged in conversation with the SlaveMaster, the slave doesn't have to enter the SlaveMaster's consciousness by saying "SlaveMaster, Sir?"

When the SlaveMaster has asked His slave a question, the slave doesn't need to ask the SlaveMaster's intention regarding making a comment.

A slave refers to other slaves as "slave," as slave (first name), "slave brother," or the Birth number of a Born slave.

"Sir, beg Your pardon, Sir" is the only way a slave expresses its accidental activities. A slave never says "sorry," or "excuse me." It would be appropriate for a slave to use "Beg Your Pardon, Sir" in a crowd when it has bumped into another.

"Sir, beg Your pardon, Sir" is also the appropriate response when a slave didn't hear or clearly understand an order. A slave says "Sir, Yes Sir, Thank You, Sir!" only when it fully understood the explanation or order and when it feels the appreciation for having it given it.

A slave enters into a conversation in the SlaveMaster's presence by asking "SlaveMaster, Sir?" "Sir, do You wish Your slave to make a comment, Sir?" This allows the slave into the conversation. The SlaveMaster might also directly invite the slave into the conversation with a sign, a word, a look, or a nod which indicates the SlaveMaster's order to speak. The slave, as always, responds "Sir, Yes Sir, Thank You, Sir!"

When speaking with the SlaveMaster, every sentence is begun and ended with the word "Sir," and EVERY pause filled with "Sir" whether for a breath, a new thought, or any other purpose. When there is more than one thought to express, the slave can use a single "Sir" between sentences so that two "Sir's" aren't expressed together. Thoughts are expressed clearly, succinctly, and without run-on. Each thought is ended, rather than held with "you know," "uh," or any other holder of speech. No holder of speech is ever used except for "Sir."

Slaves are free to speak between themselves, even in the presence of their SlaveMaster, so long as it is not distracting, does not compete with what the SlaveMaster wants to express, can be immediately and easily interrupted by the SlaveMaster interjecting, and doesn't interfere with the position the slave is currently holding. Being PRESENTED is a non-moving position. Speech is not an excuse to move.

A slave can always ask for clarification and understanding. it can ask if the SlaveMaster is ready to receive its comments, but a slave does not ever argue!

In writing, any reference to a slave is always in the small case, even at the beginning of a sentence. References to persons of respect are always capitalized. The prohibited use of I, me and my applies to writing, the same as in speech.

ORDERS

Every question a slave asks regarding the SlaveMaster's intention becomes an order once the SlaveMaster answers.

A slave PRESENTS itself to say with its presence that it has completed all orders, has no need for the SlaveMaster's attention, and is ready for the next order. When all current orders are complete, the slave comes within the SlaveMaster's line of sight, and presents itself. If the SlaveMaster is sitting or lying down, the slave presents itself in the standard way, fully PRESENTED, on its knees. When the SlaveMaster is standing, the slave has the option to PRESENT itself STANDING, but can always fully PRESENT itself whenever that is what feels natural.

Anything else may be added as is deemed important. Further, as time progresses, through its training, advice will become orders for the slave. Some of those orders will include what the slave is to do between sessions to improve its life and to prepare for slavery. Ultimately, with Birth, the control is absolute and lifelong. During the training, the orders deal with obvious improvements that should be made to prepare the slave for the responsibilities it will have after Birth.

BEHAVIOR

In general, a slave must learn and accept all slave behavior as being normal, and learns to behave in a way that feels and IS natural-looking. Additionally, the slave always acts and responds to make the SlaveMaster look "right" about the orders He gives. A slave does not respond in any way that causes the appearance that the SlaveMaster has made a mistake. This is not a game of "gotcha."

The slave is considered a part of the SlaveMaster's body. The slave is to learn to act as naturally, with the same obedience and coordination as any other part of the SlaveMaster's body. To act any other way is to act in a disabled, disrespectful and disobedient way. A slave does not invite mockery nor criticism, and feels none when it is doing as ordered. If the slave cannot accept its behavior as normal, it is unfair to expect an observer to accept it as normal. A slave always acts with dignity, and in a way that reflects positively on its Owner and its brothers.

A slave stands, no matter what the circumstance, whenever its SlaveMaster stands or He enters the same room or space as a slave. Even if the slave has been told to "stay" or to "sit," that order is only good until its SlaveMaster next enters or stands.

When told to "sit," a slave sits on the floor. That is what "sit" means to a slave. When a slave is told to "lie down," it does so on a slave mattress or pad, not a bed. Beds and chairs are furniture which a slave is not authorized to use without being specifically ordered to do so.

A slave does not sit anywhere, at any time, without the specific order of its SlaveMaster, except for in a room designated as slave space. That space may be designated within the SlaveMaster's home, or at any other location. If such a space is not designated, then a slave is NOT free to sit. Even when in the slave space, if the SlaveMaster enters that space, the slave would immediately rise to the PRESENT position, and remain in that position until told to "continue" or until given another order.

A slave never begins to eat until its SlaveMaster has begun, AND everyone due respect who is within the SlaveMaster's communication or concern has begun. A slave's authority to eat is given when the SlaveMaster authorizes food to be prepared for the slave, or when a slave is authorized to order from a menu. A slave does not ask if it is its SlaveMaster's intention for the slave to eat when there is food sitting in front of the slave, but it doesn't begin to consume that food until all, except slaves, have begun. If any Master in the area is not eating, the slave must have an explicit order to begin eating. At an eating table, a slave stands PRESENTED, rather than fully presenting while awaiting orders to sit and begin.

A slave only uses the toilet the SlaveMaster has designated for it to use, and never uses the toilet seat, nor stands in front of that toilet to piss. When a slave uses the designated toilet, or any clean, private toilet, the slave lifts the lid and seat, then sits on the rim of the seat. Afterwards, the seat and lid are lowered.

When a slave feels the need for food or drink, the slave always asks its SlaveMaster His need first, then adds, "and Your slave?" A sample behavior would include:

- PRESENTING appropriately, either full or standing
- Asking "SlaveMaster, Sir?"
- Awaiting acknowledgment
- Asking "Sir, do You wish Your slave to get You some water, Sir?"
- Responding "Sir, Yes Sir, Thank You, Sir!"
- Then adding "and Your slave, Sir?"
- Again responding "Sir, Yes Sir, Thank You, Sir!"

Whenever another slave presents, all slaves in the presence of the one who is required to PRESENT will PRESENT with that slave, i.e., a slave never watches another slave PRESENT itself, it joins the other slave in PRESENTING. Once PRESENTED, all slaves must wait for an order which allows each slave to move once again. The only exception is when the NON-PRESENTED slaves have been ordered to sleep and are in their ordered positions to sleep or when bound or otherwise encumbered in such a way that the PRESENTATION position cannot be physically achieved. PRESENTED slaves always align in an orderly fashion.

A slave walks to the left and about one step behind its SlaveMaster, with its hands behind its back. Even when walking, as always, a slave only speaks after it has requested, "SlaveMaster, Sir?" unless responding to its SlaveMaster's questions.

PUBLIC BEHAVIOR

A slave responds to its SlaveMaster's presence in public the same as in private with some modifications to prevent inviting public criticism. The slave's behavior must always engender respect for slavery, and for its SlaveMaster. No activity is to ever intentionally nor carelessly endanger that objective. Under most public circumstances, the following modification will accommodate the public's acceptance and understanding.

In the general public, a slave normally would PRESENT STANDING instead of FULLY, to enter or leave the SlaveMaster's presence.

In a restaurant, a slave stands at the end of the booth in a modified PRESENT, much like a parade rest, with the hands held open over the crack of the ass, until the SlaveMaster tells the slave, or points to the seat, to indicate that the slave should sit. The slave would discretely say "Sir, Yes Sir, Thank You, Sir!" and take its seat. When the SlaveMaster stands for any reason, the slave would again rise to the modified PRESENT STANDING position. it would enter the position gracefully and naturally, and would not look hurried, clumsy, or "put on." The slave remains in that position until the SlaveMaster issues another order. A slave stands by in the same modified PRESENT STANDING position under any circumstance within the restaurant that it would be doing so privately.

A slave refers to every man, regardless of age or position, as "Sir" at least once in every conversation. This includes check-out clerks and everyone else with whom the slave comes in contact. The only optional exception is a clearly-declared slave.

In a public or work situation around people who are not aware of the lifestyle, or where it would clearly be inappropriate, a slave does its best to avoid saying I, me and my through the use of phrases such as "One might recommend ..." or "This one would ..." A slave never uses language which would invite criticism, cause disrespect for slaves, or endanger the effectiveness of the slave's work or profession.

PROTOCOL AROUND OTHERS IN THE LIFESTYLE

Whether in public or private, a slave PRESENTS itself, in this sequence, to:

- its SlaveMaster, expressing "SlaveMaster, Sir" until told to continue or ordered otherwise.

- The Master to whom the slave has been assigned, when applicable, will be addressed as "Master, Sir" and the slave will remain until told to continue or is otherwise ordered.

- PRESENT to others by direct order. When alone, a slave PRESENTS to other knowledgeable Masters who understand the PRESENT formality, and whom the slave has previously met.

- Finally, PRESENT STANDING to each Born slave.

When a slave is with its Master, the slave's obedience is to its SlaveMaster unless its SlaveMaster directs, "Serve Your Master" at the time of presentation. Nevertheless, a slave obeys any order either its SlaveMaster or its Master issues. It is the SlaveMaster and Master's responsibility to assure there are no conflicts.

All other activity must have been satisfied, and this is done at the first opportunity that isn't distracting nor disturbing to the slave Owners. When a response has been received from the Born slave, the slave is free to continue whatever activity or circumstance it was in. Born slaves also present to each other in the same way.

Whenever anyone touches, fondles, grabs, or otherwise uses a slave without the Owner's permission, the slave respectfully says "Sir, this is the SlaveMaster's slave. Please get His permission to use it, Sir." The slave will neither indicate interest nor discouragement, nor show attitude of any form when expressing this truth.

This slave has read everything above, understands it, and agrees to accept and live by the principles listed. Failure to comply will be used only to indicate this slave's intention to immediately end this relationship, and to end its training.

SLAVES ARE BORN TO SLAVERY

An Article by SlaveMaster

Some humans are born to be slaves. Some are meant to be Born again, as slaves. There exists a natural development process that prepares a slave, and ultimately provides a Birth to slavery. The Birth of a slave "frees" it to experience all the joys, pleasures, strength and pride of slavery. The Birth is the beginning of a permanent and very legitimate life and lifestyle as a slave. Physical S/M provides the energy, along with the motivation and the "truth," that causes someone to be Born a slave. A Born slave knows, forever, that he is a slave, and never again has to remember, or be reminded, that he is one.

The special creatures meant to be slaves sense the need to serve at an early age. Others, through frustration developed over the years, know their lives just don't make sense when they aren't functioning in slavery, in service, or in a special and designated way. Some compelling internal force causes our attraction to slavery. The mores and culture of our present-day society don't, however, recognize slavery as a legitimate pursuit.

A slave is a completely separate and distinct creature on earth. It isn't a human who acts like a slave. The slave animal has characteristics unique to, and in common with, only other slaves. They possess characteristics which aren't (and can't be) trained into someone, but which are present in all who have been Born a slave. Training only discovers the slave within; it doesn't create it or define it.

A lack of understanding or knowledge of the true nature and existence of these special animals, who are slaves and no longer human, has caused those meant to be slaves to seek and submit to all sorts of experiences. Some have been fortunate to find a caring Master who has instincts about the potential and value of a slave. Many have exposed themselves to very unfulfilling or dangerous circumstances that don't develop who a slave really is.

This is about the real and complete process by which someone permanently gives up being a human to be something better, BEING BORN A SLAVE. This is for those for whom "acting" like a slave is not enough. This is the process by which either novice or well-trained slaves find their full, final identity that distinguishes them from the people in the world, and supplies them with invincible self-esteem that is virtually unequaled by others.

Slavery Birth is a natural growth process based on S/M that redefines who someone is, how they think and how they live. Just like being gay, some are born to their genetic parents, meant to grow up and destined to be slave. To become a slave animal, replacing the human animal, it is necessary to be Born a second time. This time, however, there is only one "parent," i.e., the SlaveMaster. Just as you can have only one natural father, a slave can only be Born to one person who is forever its Owner. The relationship formed at Birth between a slave and his SlaveMaster is life-long. The Birth is no less eventful and dramatic than the original genetic birth. This slave training and Birth process is the ultimate step for someone serious enough about him- or herself and their slavery, honest enough with themselves to accept who they are, and courageous enough to do something about it.

Born slavery is for those whose lives are incomplete without the permanence of slavery. There are some very good "performance" slaves in this world. These slaves, through mutual consent or by contract, have agreed to take on and accept a role of slavery. Those who take the role seriously allow their attitudes to change over time and to become slave-like. That makes someone valuable and worth owning. Performance slavery probably plays a valuable place in our S/M society. It allows for slavery that can be on-again, off-again. It allows for Masters to take a slave and abandon him at will. It allows for slavery one night at a time. Some slaves want to confine their activity to predetermined circumstances such as these. Certainly, no criticism is intended for such slaves. Anyone who is willing to accept the role of a slave, under any circumstance, is worthy of note. Such humans are very endearing, and typically very caring and pleasurable individuals.

When someone is Born, however, it gives up being human. He becomes something far superior to who he was when burdened with human limitations; he becomes SLAVE. A slave cannot become slave without someone to be a slave to, just as no child can be born without parents. A Born slave is Born to his SlaveMaster. A SlaveMaster cannot be a SlaveMaster without slaves, and a slave cannot be a slave without a SlaveMaster. It must be a permanent and continuing connection, and it is even more critical than a child's relationship to his parents. It is far more intimate, and a slave never outgrows the connection. The benefits continue to expand over time. Similarly, no matter what a child does with and during his life, his security, identity and strength continue to be derived from his or her parents, with knowledge of their love and support throughout life. For a slave, the SlaveMaster is that continuous source of strength and guidance, and much more!

A Born slave lives every second of its life with the self-image of "slave." The slave's security comes from having a "family" to which it will always belong. Some performance slaves are lucky enough to have long-term Masters. They can develop the same sense of self-identity over time, but still can be sold, exchanged, or simply dropped if the Master so decides.

By comparison, a SlaveMaster owns the slave for so long as He lives. A Born slave may be assigned by his SlaveMaster to serve another, who becomes his Master, but he serves the Master in service to his SlaveMaster. More completely than owning property, a slave is owned in the

229

same way that the SlaveMaster owns His own hand. A slave is a part of the SlaveMaster's body.

Every aspect of the connection between a slave and his SlaveMaster is absolutely and identically the same as that between a man and his body. The slave takes its identity from its SlaveMaster. The SlaveMaster expects the same obedience from His slave that He does from His hand, and as He would from any part of His body. The SlaveMaster cares for and identifies with the slave, as He does His own hand, and would never do anything with His hand, or His slave, that is not in its best interest.

Likewise, the slave provides his SlaveMaster with information, just as the SlaveMaster's hand would provide information that the hand receives. However, in the same way as a slave, the hand would not, and cannot, question what a Man does with His own hand. Nor is the hand functional if given away. The bond and the connection are permanent, and for life.

When slaves are Born, their purpose and destiny in life are made clear. It is part of the gift of slavery. Two of the first three slaves Born to me were assigned to other men, their Masters. Those two slaves have lived with those Men, and have been Their slaves. It is what was meant to happen for those slaves at the time of their Birth. However, life's circumstances can and do change over time, and what is to be done with each who is a Born slave is different for each slave.

A SlaveMaster is on the same side as His slave and must know what He is doing. He controls His slave's life. Where a Man and His Born slave stand together, only one Man stands. A slave is part of his SlaveMaster in every way. Each order must, therefore, reflect the best interest of the slave, because a slave can never disobey any order. A slave's Birth is achievable only because of an internally-sworn obedience that has no qualifications, no time limits and no exceptions. If a slave cannot offer such obedience, it will never be Born. A SlaveMaster must take that responsibility very, very seriously. In Birth, a slave experiences his SlaveMaster's intention directly and knows that he can trust that He will take it seriously, and so offers his obedience without reluctance.

It is because of this unquestioned control that a SlaveMaster will never be found to have only one slave. The human tendency to let personal needs interfere with the best interest of an only slave, who has sworn unqualified obedience, is too great. Objectivity is possible only when there are alternatives to satisfying the personal needs of a Man who has absolute authority over others.

At Birth, a slave is given the power needed to fulfill his purpose and, at the same time, such a strong sense of self-esteem and self-identity that he never needs to look inward again. When a man knows who he is and what his purpose is, that provides him the freedom to have single focus, full-time devotion to his only purpose, which is service in slavery. That service could include any profession, any variety of relationship, devotion to genetic "blood," relatives, friendships, satisfaction of social obligations, and many other forms of service.

Born slavery is not an escape. It is the putting of oneself in the position that he must obey all orders to do what should be done, without option or argument. It is a letting-go of the right to decide to fail. Success in every area of life becomes a requirement, not an option.

- **WHAT IS THE ACTUAL PROCESS OF BEING BORN TO SLAVERY?**

It begins with an honest commitment from a potential Born slave to explore the reality of who he really is. The Birth experience itself is dramatic and spiritual, and it occurs at a specific date and time in which the permanent union takes place between a slave and his SlaveMaster.

The Birth process makes it clear that slavery is how it must live, and that being a slave is all that he is. The experience is so intense, so real, and so enlightening, that the truth can never again be denied. Until Birth, a slave is still only a potential slave because he has the option of not becoming a Born slave. After Birth, that option is not a reasonable one. The denial would have to be so intense that it would have serious adverse impact on a man's life who is trying not to live as a slave after truly discovering and knowing he is a slave.

Slave training, then, must be an intense and exacting process. A man must be forced to examine everything he believes, and examine his willingness to obey one man always. This obedience will be without qualification or limitation, for the rest of his life. He must be dedicated to a life of absolute honesty, without the option or opportunity to play "people games" like manipulation ever again. The option of self-control is lost once and for always. These are soul-searching questions and commitments that, unsatisfied, prevent Birth.

The gift of slavery does not provide any escape from reality. It is not a place to hide, or run from responsibilities. It does just the opposite. It makes the slavery real, and forces it into the world around us, to serve it and the people in it. It takes away the option not to develop and live in a way that fulfills destiny, according to its plan and place in the universe.

The SlaveMaster's responsibility is to support everything a slave is intended to do with his life professionally, socially, in relationship and all ways that are revealed during Birth. His responsibility is also to the continued growth and health of the slavery itself, apart from and beyond the one who is the slave. Hence the title, "SlaveMaster."

• WHAT IS A BORN SLAVE?

When a man or woman is Born, a new identity, with its own energy and personality, comes to life. The human must step aside and let the mind, body, heart and soul that he has been using for years, be given completely and irreversibly to his SlaveMaster.

A slave's ego is used only to care for the SlaveMaster's slave when he is away from his SlaveMaster. When he is with his SlaveMaster, all thoughts, feelings and sensations are given to the SlaveMaster and used as the SlaveMaster sees fit. Nothing belongs to the slave, except the slavery itself, and his SlaveMaster.

The slave spirit is always available to guide the slave through life, as by instinct. At the time of Birth, and whenever a slave's SlaveMaster returns him to his spiritual place of Birth, only the pure slave spirit is present. At those times, there is no evidence of the man who once lived in the body of the slave. That pure slave spirit will only appear when special circumstances are present.

To begin with, a slave spirit exists only when no conscious activity is present or required. If a slave attempts to form a single English word, even as simple as "yes" or "no," the spirit vanishes. If a slave is required to make a dichotomous (either/or) decision about whether he is to do this or that, the spirit disappears. If a slave is given an order that is unclear, the conscious question about what to do will cause the spirit to go away. It is very particular about the environment in which it will exist. Therefore, the SlaveMaster has no option about what environment must be provided during the training to allow for Birth.

A slave spirit will appear only when it knows that its obedience is so complete that if the slave man receives a feeling and is ordered by his SlaveMaster differently, the slave will obey rather than follow the internal feeling.

Without that extreme level of trust, where the Owner is trusted more than self, the spirit is not safe to appear.

When a man abandons himself, he needs to know that there is someone whom he will absolutely obey who is watching and caring for him even more intensely than he cares for himself.

Without that level of confidence, the spirit considers it too dangerous to appear. Absolute obedience is therefore a minimum requirement. The obedience needs to be so complete that even the thought of taking back control is not as much of a possibility. That obedience is the parachute that allows jumping out of the slave spirit "airplane." Without a parachute, the process is mentally suicidal, and will never happen.

When a man, however, has abandoned himself and only the slave is present, that is the pure slave state. When in the slave state, several characteristics are commonly witnessed.

First, there is a tremendous sense of power and peace, a sense of being connected to the universe and not alone, a part of everything that is happening in the world. After the original Birth, when taken back by his SlaveMaster, being in that state lowers the heart rate to about half, breathing to less than half, blood pressure so low that the slave must be in the reclined position and minimally bound because there isn't sufficient pressure to supply blood to the other side of the bondage.

Another experience of being in the pure state of slavery is that all thoughts in the room, and the location of everyone in the room who produces those thoughts, are clear. Even being fully- hooded and ear-plugged doesn't affect the information a slave is given. The most universal characteristic of being in the slave state, however, is that the slave can feel no pain. No matter what is done to the slave in the slave state, every touch of a flogger or whip, or any device, is interpreted in a positive way. It is viewed as power, love, belonging, meaning, insight and many other varied things, different and dependent on each experience. Being in the slave state is not an escape from the physical discipline. The slave feeds on it, needs it and wants it.

It is a SlaveMaster's responsibility to return a slave to his slave state periodically to provide the nourishment a slave needs to maintain his rarified, special, and unique existence. For a Born slave, it takes only from 10-15 minutes to return to that state at the hand and physical discipline of his SlaveMaster, to whom he was Born. There is nothing tricky or clever needed. For the SlaveMaster, it is an automatic "walk-in the-park" process that requires nothing but the intention to do so.

Being returned to that place of Birth, to the pure slave state, is probably the greatest reward of true, Born slavery. It provides a slave with the unique abilities and experiences that allow it to serve as no human could. During that special time, the slave is replenished, empowered, reconnected, enlightened and strengthened; made proud and powerful, insightful and wise. A slave is freed from all human limitations and restraints, freed from ordinary rules and the need to think and to be responsible, so that he can be prepared for the next step in his life. A slave can be granted extraordinary experiences on a regular basis. Some men have dedicated their lives to the pursuit of having such an intense experience even one time. A Born slave can assume such experiences, at the discretion of his SlaveMaster, the man to whom he owes his Birth.

The slave is taught to "present" (on knees spread apart, wrists held behind the back, head bowed) himself, when he enters his SlaveMaster's presence, and to request intention when he leaves it. The control needs to be absolute, every second, whenever in the SlaveMaster's presence. It is necessary because the slave must habitually know that he is always being controlled completely, in every action, whenever with his Owner, the SlaveMaster. A slave in training must know that he is under his SlaveMaster's control at every moment so that he can assume that to be true when Born, or afterwards, when returned to the slave state. That constant control will eventually allow the trust that is necessary for Birth to occur. During training, the slave can never be in doubt about when he is to make a decision, or when it is his Owner's decision.

Most readers will already know the human body can only sense pressure and temperature. Pain and pleasure are the brain's interpretations. The same pressure applied through physical S/M can be interpreted by a man being trained to slavery as either pain or pleasure, based on his beliefs and what he needs to experience to be Born. Physically, the slave must be exposed to "edge" physical discipline, pressures that exceed his ability to handle it. To be able to "handle" physical S/M, all the pressure a slave is exposed to implies that the man is maintaining control. The trainee must be forced to experience pressure beyond what he can handle, beyond what he can control, so that the control is transferred to another, his SlaveMaster. It forces the slave's mental processes to occur below the conscious level, at the subconscious level where what a man must experience, abandon, acknowledge, or let go of, is known. The training process is not about a slave learning to control more pressure. It's about learning not to control at all! It's about learning to let someone else, his SlaveMaster, do all the controlling. It is very different from the "slow start, transition, mind space/other side" common in S/M "play."

A SlaveMaster is not watching the slave being disciplined to determine where it is mentally, so that he can supply the right experience at the right time. The S/M sequence, the pressure, the intensity is directed from the "outside," not by the slave. The "bottom" is still in control if he is being watched for clues. That is, of course, where those silly stories about how the "slave" controls come from. It may be true for a bottom in a pure S/M experience, but not for a slave, either Born or in training to be Born. A slave knows it does not control.

In fact, it would be an extremely fearful thought for a Born slave or trainee to believe that he did control. It would be so fearful that it would prevent Birth, or return to the state of Birth. Being in control would leave no one to protect and guide it when he yields to his pure slavery. A slave would become dangerously adrift.

There are no games being played here! A slave is whole only because of the absolute will of his SlaveMaster. The last thing a slave would want, would be to be without that will. A SlaveMaster is whole only because of the absolute, unquestioned obedience of his slave. A body is considered dysfunctional when its Owner cannot depend on the obedience of His body parts, including His slaves. Likewise, when a body part, a slave included, cannot depend on the direction of its Owner, the body is dysfunctional.

Being Born to slavery is not an easy process. A man is asked to yield everything he ever was, is, or wants to be, to another Man. He is asked to live in the body of another Man who owns it, and to give every feeling, emotion, every sensation to its rightful Owner, without question, and to invite every experience, no matter what it might be. He or she is required to give up the possibility of ever being dishonest again, or to hide anything as small as a thought from its Owner. He is required to use the identity of another, alone, without any of his own, and to possess only one part of himself, his slavery. All credit or criticism for what it does is expected to be turned over to another. He is expected to cherish, cling to and protect his slavery at all costs, because it is everything he is and all that he will be. No other alternatives, no bridges, no escape routes remain. Every past experience, and bad "tape" is open to review at intense physical moments. The hope of self-control is dissolved forever. A Born slave trainee is mentally asked to sign one, final, blank check for his life and everything that will happen until the end of it.

The training is a powerful, often disturbing, always real experience. It isn't an erotic cascade of sexual events unhampered by real life. It is a pleasurable experience, otherwise no one would return even for the second session! Still, only the finest, the truest, and the best in the world "survive" all the experiences, and are Born. That is why they are so rare, and to be cherished.

The process itself can be divided into two phases. The first phase is the first four to six sessions. During that time the subconscious gets a clue, that in lock-step fashion, the ego is on a destructive course. The SlaveMaster is identified as its mortal enemy by the end of this first phase. All potential slaves ask, therefore, for a time to pause and reflect at the end of phase one. Some don't have the courage to continue, usually because of the integrity issues that it is clear will become a requirement. For the dedicated, a renewed commitment is made to continue, one more session, into phase two.

The second phase ends in Birth, but the number of sessions varies, based on the human "junk" that must be disposed of before a man can pass through the "eye of the needle" to slavery. Phase two normally takes from six to fifteen sessions after phase one has ended.

Students of slavery will recognize some of the mentality that has been discussed here. Slavery is a real state of existence. Those who are experienced and honest about being slaves, or who have had the chance to be in a performance slave position to a Master over time, have intuitively come to feel some of the "truth" about slavery. A Born slave lives that truth and has no option to live in any other way.

Being Born a slave is far more than knowledge and experience of what a slave does. Being Born is who you are! A Born slave must give up being human to accept the gift of slavery. It has been said that the good things in life are the mortal enemies of the best things in life. When we consider our slavery or our slave experiences adequate, there is little incentive to do more, to risk what we already have. A Born slave is bound to do what it must for the rest of his life, regardless of the consequences. That is a fearful and too-scary place to be, for many.

Only slave Birth, however, for those genetically born to be slaves, can give someone the full feeling that he or she is doing with his life exactly and completely what he should be doing with it. Regardless of the spiritual background, there is a sense of fulfillment, or lack of it, from what we do with our lives. For those with the courage, the dedication, and the willingness to risk, there is an answer to living fully- integrated in slavery. That answer is Birth.

There are no finer creatures on earth than those Born slaves. They are creatures you can trust implicitly, who are incapable of selfish or malicious thought. They have as their only purpose to make this planet a better one. Slaves are not made, they are not contracted, they are Born!

- **WHO IS A CANDIDATE FOR TRAINING FOR BIRTH?**

Whether or not someone is currently in a relationship, including slavery or Mastery, makes no difference. If that relationship is the right one, being Born will make it a better one. How much experience in slavery or S/M makes no difference, nor does currently having an interest in slavery matter. A willingness to explore and accept the truth is all that is required. Training is based on having mutual interest after a detailed interview. A trainee's commitment can only be to one session at a time, and few if any demands are made for what happens between sessions, until Birth. The truth that a potential Born slave is exposed to during the training causes all the personal adjustment anyone can handle until Birth provides the wisdom and power to do what should be done on a continuous basis.

Some haven't considered being slaves because of the poor misconceptions that many have about slaves and slavery. Candidates include those who feel they are unsatisfied no matter what they do or try or what kind of relationships they get into. Candidates also include those who feel that only progressively more extreme experiences can provide satisfaction. If happiness isn't a gift of your current slavery, then the "something more" you might be lacking may be Born slavery.

About The BornSlaves Group
A final note from SlaveMaster

www.BornSlaves.com

I'm impressed and excited by the membership and participation in this group. I'm encouraged by both the number of Master/Owners and slaves, and the depth of their commitment to the spiritual path. Looking for, wanting, working for and accepting a legitimate position in life greater than the entertainment of our fetishes is rewarding and challenging, and this group's membership reflects the desire and willingness to make an investment of time and effort to achieve more than what being a "player" brings.

I personally have neither a spiritual nor a psychological academic background. I make no attempt to explain nor justify anything based on any theory or discipline. What I know, I know through experience, or through My own unwavering obedience. I'm neither defensive about, nor do I take personally, any comments or objections to the Truth I've been given. I'm merely passing on what has been passed to Me, for purposes I am not meant to know. The Truth affects people it is supposed to affect, and those for whom it is not intended won't "get it" until they're ready exactly as the Universe intends. The Universe doesn't ask my advice, so I'm neither consulted nor advised about what ITs intention is. I feel blessed simply to be given what I'm personally meant to know and do.

Every comment I make comes from my obedient position in life, which began with a defining moment in which I swore to never believe anything I wasn't willing to live by, and to live by everything I believe. When what I express has meaning to you, it is meant to have. When it doesn't, then it's not yet meant to have meaning for you.

The objective of this site is for each of us to provide beliefs that both apply now and that will apply in the future when we're ready for that belief. I ask that we avoid frustration from not seeing it all now. To a child, a parent leaving it with a babysitter to go to the store can look like abandonment. As the beliefs change through experience, that same child will eventually recognize the gift of the parent leaving to acquire what it needs. The action is the same, but the understanding and perspective change.

It is therefore important to express what you believe now, without concern for its acceptance. Telling the truth will help others understand where you are and will better assist them in facilitating their growth. Those who do not understand haven't reached the same place yet, but are better prepared to accept and recognize the lesson when it does come. Either way, no comment is to be taken personally. It is assumed that each posting is intended only to serve the others in the group, and it is not the promulgation of a personal agenda. This is what I have already observed here, and it is as I hoped it would be.

My best to you all,

SlaveMaster

ABOUT US:

Known by the spiritual name of **SlaveMaster**, he hails from the Pacific Northwest, where he held the Portland Mr. Leather and Pacific Northwest Mr. Leather titles. He currently lives in Nevada. He participates in BDSM and Master/slave events throughout the nation. He was actively involved in the Butchmann's Experience, conducted in various cities throughout the U.S.

Developing slaves' destiny has been his focus for over two decades. SlaveMaster regards slavery as a legitimate, admirable calling, and believes it is his privilege and purpose in life to bring slaves to Birth. Finding those who are His slaves is as important to Him as it is for His slaves to find Him. An open invitation exists to any who believe they are destined to be owned.

Email: SlaveMaster@BornSlaves.com

slave 7 — so named due to his Birth order — is an educator and musician. Although originally from California, he states he has now found authentic living in the desert of Nevada. He is "a friend of what is natural and honest, but no friend of the ego."   He believes that finding new ways every day to be obedient is what life is about, and what gives it meaning.

Email: SMslave7@Yahoo.com

Summer Sterling is the author of "Confessions of a Bad Submissive," and "No Pain, No Gain," available at www.PinkFlamingo.com, www.EroticBookNetwork.com, as well as other major outlets. She is a writer of BDSM erotica; memoir, and award-winning essays under various pen names. She is heavily involved in animal rescue; cooking, organic gardening and natural beekeeping. Her greatest joy is serving her tremendously wise and supportive husband.

Email: SummerSterling2015@gmail.com